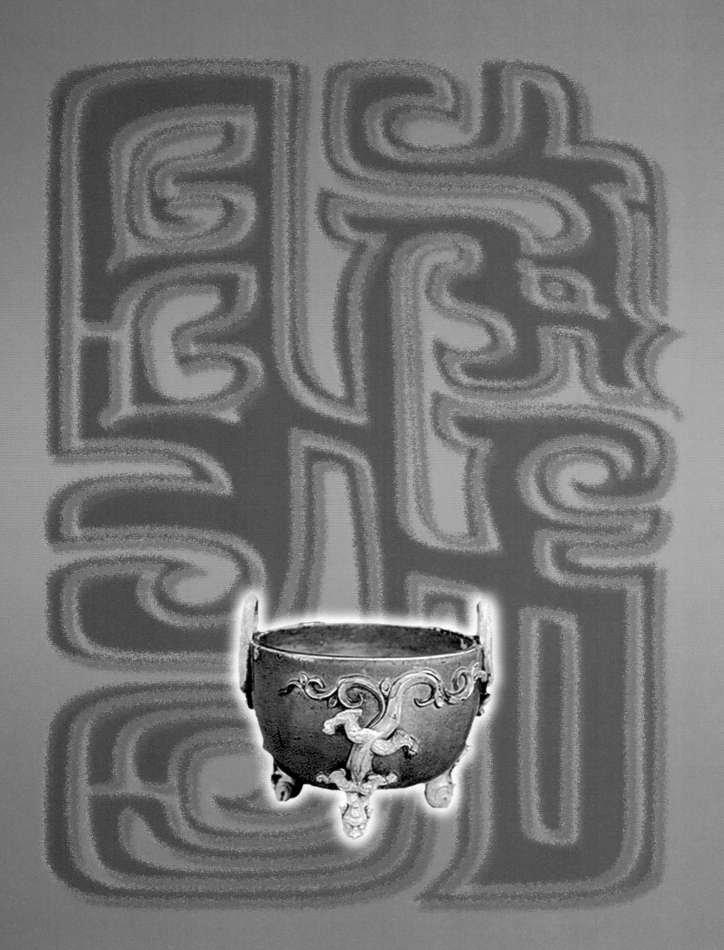

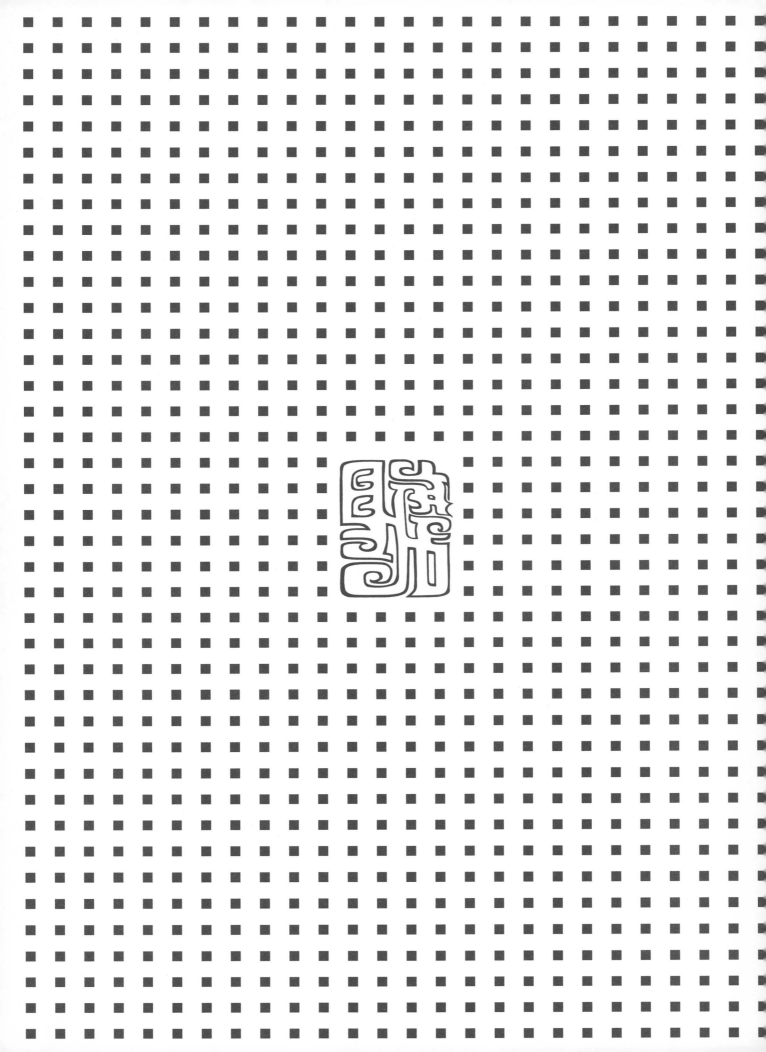

国家出版基金项目
NATIONAL PUBLICATION FOUNDATION

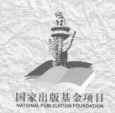

中华医药卫生

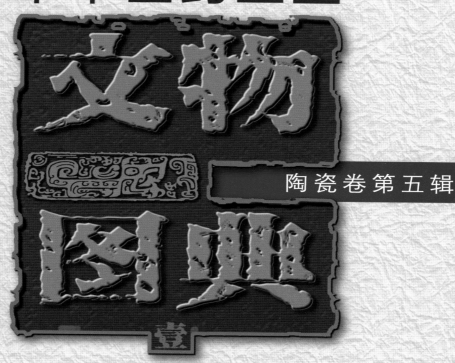

陶瓷卷第五辑

主　编　李经纬　梁　峻　刘学春
总主译　白永权
主　译　范晓晖　温　睿

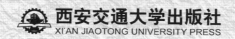

西安交通大学出版社
XI'AN JIAOTONG UNIVERSITY PRESS

图书在版编目（CIP）数据

中华医药卫生文物图典 . 1 . 陶瓷卷 . 第 5 辑 . / 李经纬，
梁峻，刘学春主编 . — 西安：西安交通大学出版社，2016.12

ISBN 978-7-5605-7032-7

Ⅰ . ①中… Ⅱ . ①李… ②梁… ③刘… Ⅲ . ①中国医药学—
古代陶瓷—中国—图录 Ⅳ . ① R-092 ② K870.2

中国版本图书馆 CIP 数据核字（2015）第 013563 号

书　　名	中华医药卫生文物图典（一）陶瓷卷第五辑
主　　编	李经纬　梁　峻　刘学春
责任编辑	张沛烨

出版发行	西安交通大学出版社
	（西安市兴庆南路 10 号　邮政编码 710049）
网　　址	http://www.xjtupress.com
电　　话	（029）82668805　82668502（医学分社）
	（029）82668315（总编办）
传　　真	（029）82668280
印　　刷	中煤地西安地图制印有限公司

开　　本	889mm×1194mm　1/16　　印张 21　字数 328 千字
版次印次	2017 年 12 月第 1 版　2017 年 12 月第 1 次印刷
书　　号	ISBN 978-7-5605-7032-7
定　　价	680.00 元

读者购书、书店添货、如发现印装质量问题，请通过以下方式联系、调换。

订购热线：（029）82665248　（029）82665249

投稿热线：（029）82668805　（029）82668502

读者信箱：medpress@126.com

铭记感受历史

自信自重自强

中华医药卫生文场图典问世

书贺

陈可冀 谨题

二〇一七年清月

陈可冀　中国科学院院士、国医大师

精修醫藥衛生文物

圖典功著當代

深究岐黃學術思想

淵源惠澤千秋

中華醫藥衛生文物圖典出版誌慶

丁酉孟秋 孫光榮 敬題於北京

孫光榮　国医大师

中華醫藥衛生文物圖典出版

彰顯中醫藥
文化精神

體現中醫藥
歷史價值

歲次丁酉夏　王琦

王琦　国医大师

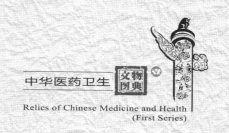

中华医药卫生
Relics of Chinese Medicine and Health
(First Series)

中华医药卫生文物图典（一）
丛书编撰委员会

主　编　李经纬　梁　峻　刘学春

副主编　廖　果　吴鸿洲　康兴军　和中浚　刘小斌　杨金生

　　　　　郑怀林　徐江雁　白建疆　黄　煌

编　委　李洪晓　梁永宣　王强虎　董树平　马　健　王　霞

　　　　　张雅宗　朱德明　包哈申　张建青　郑　蓉　庄乾竹

　　　　　李宏红　刘哲峰　王宏才　陈润东

总主译　白永权

主　译　陈向京　聂文信　范晓晖　温　睿　赵永生　杜彦龙

　　　　　吉　乐　李小棉　郭　梦　陈　曦

副主译（按姓氏音序排列）

　　　　　董艳云　姜雨孜　李建西　刘　慧　马　健　任宝磊

　　　　　任　萌　任　莹　王　颇　习通源　谢皖吉　徐素云

　　　　　许崇钰　许　梅　詹菊红　赵　菲　邹郝晶

译　者（按姓氏音序排列）

迟征宇　邓　甜　付一豪　高　琛　高　媛　郭　宁

韩　蕾　何宗昌　胡勇强　黄　鋆　蒋新蕾　康晓薇

李静波　刘雅恬　刘妍萌　鲁显生　马　月　牛笑语

唐云鹏　唐臻娜　田　多　铁红玲　佟健一　王　晨

王　丹　王　栋　王　丽　王　媛　王慧敏　王梦杰

王仙先　吴耀均　席　慧　肖国强　许子洋　闫红贤

杨姣姣　姚　晔　张　阳　张　鋆　张继飞　张梦原

张晓谦　赵　欣　赵亚力　郑　青　郑艳华　朱江嵩

朱瑛培

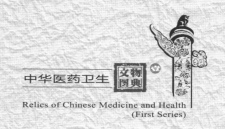

中华医药卫生 文物图典

Relics of Chinese Medicine and Health
(First Series)

本册编撰委员会

主　编　李经纬　梁　峻　刘学春

副主编　廖　果　吴鸿洲　康兴军　和中浚　刘小斌　杨金生
　　　　郑怀林　徐江雁　白建疆　黄　煌

编　委　李洪晓　梁永宣　王强虎　董树平　马　健　王　霞
　　　　张雅宗　朱德明　包哈申　张建青　郑　蓉　庄乾竹
　　　　李宏红　刘哲峰　王宏才　陈润东

总主译　白永权

主　译　范晓晖　温　睿

副主译　马　健　习通源

译　者　李静波　张　鋆　肖国强　赵　菲　马　月

丛书策划委员会

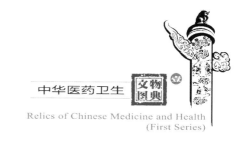

中华医药卫生 文物图典

Relics of Chinese Medicine and Health
(First Series)

序 言

　　探索天、地、人运动变化规律以及"气化物生"过程的相互关系，是人类永恒的课题。宇宙不可逆，地球不可逆，人生不可逆业已成为共识。天地造化形成自然，人类活动构成文化。文物既是文化的载体，又是物化的历史，还是文明的见证。

　　追求健康长寿是人类共同的夙愿。中华民族之所以繁衍昌盛，健康文化起了巨大的推动作用。由于古人谋求生存发展、应对环境变化产生的智慧，大多反映在以医药卫生为核心的健康文化之中，所以，习总书记说："中医药学是中国古代科学的瑰宝，也是打开中华文明宝库的钥匙"。

　　秉持文化大发展、大繁荣理念，中国中医科学院李经纬、梁峻等为负责人的科研团队在完成科技部"国家重点医药卫生文物收集调研和保护"课题获 2005 年度中华中医药学会科技二等奖基础上，又资鉴"夏商周断代工程""中华文明探源工程"等相关考古成果，用有重要价值的新出土文物置换原拍摄质量较差的文物，适当补充民族医药文物，共精选收载 5000 余件。经西安交通大学出版社申报，《中华医药卫生文物图典（一）》（以下简称《图典》）于 2013 年获得了国家出版基金的资助，并经专业翻译团队翻译，使《图典》得以面世。

　　文物承载的信息多元丰富，发掘解读其中蕴藏的智慧并非易事。医药卫生文物更具有特殊性，除文物的一般属性外，还承载着传统医学发展史迹与促进健康的信息。运用历史唯物主义观察发掘文物信息，善于从生活文物中领悟卫生信息，才能准确解读其功能，也才能诠释其在民生健康中的历史作用，收到以古鉴今之效果。"历史是现实的根源"，任何一个民族都不能割断历史，史料都包含在文化中。"文化是民族的血脉，是人民的精神家园"，文化繁荣才能实现中华民族的伟大复兴。值本《图典》付梓之际，用"梳理文化之脉，必获健康之果"作为序言并和作者、读者共勉！

中央文史研究馆馆员

中国工程院院士　　王永炎

丁酉年仲夏

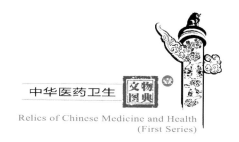

中华医药卫生 文物图典

Relics of Chinese Medicine and Health
(First Series)

前 言

　　文化是相对自然的概念，是考古界常用词汇。文物是文化的重要组成部分，既是文明的物证，又是物化的历史。狭义医药卫生文物是疾病防治模式语境下的解读，而广义医药卫生文物则是躯体、心态、环境适应三维健康模式下的诠释。中华民族是 56 个民族组成的多元一体大家庭，中华医药卫生文物当然包括各民族的健康文化遗存。

　　天地造化如造山、板块漂移、气候变迁、生物起源进化等形成自然。气化物生莫贵于人，即整个生物进化的最高成果是人类自身。广义而言，人类生存思维留下的痕迹即物质财富和精神财富总和构成文化，其一般的物化形式是视觉感知的文物、文献、胜迹等。其中质变标志明晰的文化如文字、文物、城市、礼仪等可称作文明。从唯物史观视角观察，狭义文化即精神财富，尤其体现人类精、气、神状态的事项，其本质也具有特殊物质属性，如量子也具有波粒二相性，这种粒子也是物质，无非运动方式特殊而已。现代所谓可重复验证的"科学"，事实上也是从文化中分离出来的事项，因此也是一种特殊文化形式。追求健康长寿是人类共同的夙愿。中华民族之所以繁衍昌盛，是因为健康文化异彩纷呈。中华优秀传统医药文化之所以博大精深，是因为其原创思维博大、格物致知精深，所以，习总书记说："中医药学是中国古代科学的瑰宝，也是打开中华文明宝库的钥匙"。

文化既反映时代、地域、民族分布、生产资料来源、技术水平等信息，又反映人类认知水平和生存智慧。发掘解读文物、文献中蕴藏的健康知识和灵动智慧，首先是从事健康工作者的责任和义务。《易经》设有"观"卦，人类作为观察者，不仅要积极收藏展陈文物，而且要善于捕捉文物倾诉的信息，汲取养分，启迪思维，收到古为今用之效果。墨子三表法，首先一表即"本之于古者圣王之事"，也是强调古代史实的重要性。"历史是现实的根源"，现实是未来的基础。任何一个国家、地区、民族都不能割断历史、忽略基础，这个基础就是文化。"文化是民族的血脉，是人民的精神家园"。文化繁荣才能驱动各项事业发展，才能实现中华民族的伟大复兴。

人类从类人猿分化出来。"禄丰古猿禄丰种"是云南禄丰发现的类人猿化石，距今七八百万年。距今200万年前人类进入旧石器时代，直立行走，打制石器产生工具意识，管理火种，是所谓"燧人氏"时代。中国留存有更新世早、中期的元谋、蓝田、北京人等遗址。距今10万—5万年前，人类进入旧石器时代中期，即早期智人阶段，脑容量增加，和欧洲、非洲人种相比，原始蒙古人种颧骨前突等，是所谓"伏羲氏"时代。中国发现的马坝、长阳、丁村人等较典型。距今5万—1万年前，人类进入旧石器时代晚期，即晚期智人阶段，细石器、骨角器等遍布全国，山顶洞、柳江、资阳人等较典型。

中石器时代距今约1万年，是旧石器时代向新石器时代的短暂过渡期，弓箭发明，狗被驯化。河南灵井、陕西沙苑遗址等作为代表。距今1万—公元前2600年前后，人类进入新石器时代，磨光石器、烧制陶器，出现农业村落并饲养家畜，是所谓"神农氏"时代。公元前7000年以来，在甲、骨、陶、石等载体上出现契刻符号、七音阶骨笛乐器等，反映出人文气息趋浓。公元前6000—公元前3500年的老官台、裴李岗、河姆渡、马家浜、仰韶等文化遗址，彰显出先民围绕生存健康问题所做的各种努力。

公元前4800年以来，以关中、晋南、豫西为中心形成的仰韶文化，是中原史前文化的重要标志。以半坡、庙底沟类型为典型，自公元前3500年走向繁荣，属于锄耕粟黍稻兼营渔猎饲养猪鸡经济方式，彩陶尤其发达。公元前4400—公元前3300年，长江中游的大溪文化，薄胎彩陶和白陶发达。公元前4300—公元前2500年山东丰岛的大汶口文化，红陶为主。公元前3500年前后，辽东的红山文化原始宗教发展。公元前 3300 年以来，长江下游由河姆渡、马家浜文化衍续的良渚文化和陇西的马家窑文化、江淮间的薛家岗文化时趋发达。

公元前 2600—公元前 2000 年，黄河中下游龙山文化群形成，冶铸铜器，制作玉器，土坯、石灰、夯筑技术开始应用。公元前 2697 年，轩辕战败炎帝（有说其后裔）、蚩尤而为黄帝纪元元年。黄帝西巡访贤，"至岐见岐伯，引载而归，访于治道"。其引归地"溱洧襟带于前，梅泰环拱于后"，即今河南新密市古城寨。岐黄答问，构建《黄帝内经》健康知识体系，中华文明从关注民生健康起步。颛顼改革宗教，神职人员出现；帝喾修身节用，帝尧和合百国，舜同律度量衡，大禹疏导治水，中华民族不断繁衍昌盛。

公元前 2070 年，禹之子启以豫西晋南为中心建立夏王朝，二里头青铜文化为其特征，半地穴、窑洞、地面建筑并存。饮食卫生器具、酒器增多。朱砂安神作用在宫殿应用。公元前 1600 年，商灭夏。偃师商城设有铸铜作坊。公元前 1300 年，盘庚迁殷，使用甲骨文。武丁时期青铜浑铸、分铸并存。公元前 1056 年，相传周"文王被殷纣拘于羑里，演《周易》，成六十四卦"。公元前 1046 年，武王克商建周，定都镐京。青铜器始铸长篇铭文，周原发掘出微型甲骨文字。公元前 770 年，平王东迁。虢国铸铜柄铁剑。公元前 753 年，秦国设置史官。公元前 707 年出现蝗灾、公元前 613 年出现"哈雷彗星"，均被孔子载入《春秋》。公元前 221 年，秦始皇统一中国，多元一体民族大家庭形成，中华医药卫生文物异彩纷呈。

中国是治史大国，历来重视发展文化博物事业，1955 年成立卫生部中医研究院时就设置医史研究室，1982 年中国医史文献研究所成立时复建中国医史博物馆研究收藏展陈文物。2000—2003 年，经王永炎院士、姚乃礼院长等呼吁，科技部批准立项，由李经纬、梁峻为负责人的团队完成"国家重点医药卫生文物收集调研和保护"项目任务，受到科技部项目验收组专家的高度评价，获中华中医药学会科技进步二等奖。2013 年，在国家出版基金资助下，课题组对部分文物重新拍摄或必要置换、充实民族医药文物后，由西安交通大学出版社编辑、组聘国内一流翻译团队英译说明文字付梓，受到国家中医药博物馆筹备工作领导小组和办公室的高度重视。

"物以类聚"，《图典》主要依据文物质地、种类分为 9 卷，计有陶瓷，金属，纸质，竹木，玉石、织品及标本，壁画石刻及遗址，少数民族文物，其他，备考等卷。同卷下主要根据历史年代或小类分册设章。每卷下的历史时段不求统一。遵循上述规则将《图典》划分为 21 册，总计收载文物 5000 余件。对每件文物的描述，除质地、规格、馆藏等基本要素外，重点描述其在民生健康中的作用。对少数暂不明确的事项在括号中注明待考。对引自各博物馆的材料除在文物后列出馆藏外，还在书后再次统一列出馆名或参考书目，以充分尊重其馆藏权，也同时维护本典作者的引用权。

21 世纪，围绕人类健康的生命科学将飞速发展，但科学离不开文化，文化离不开文物。发掘文物承载的信息为现实服务，谨引用横渠先生四言之两语："为天地立心，为生民立命"，既作为编撰本《图典》之宗旨，也是我们践行国家"一带一路"倡议的具体努力。希冀通过本《图典》的出版发行，教育国人，提振中华民族精神；走向世界，为人类健康事业贡献力量。

李经纬　梁峻　刘学春

2017 年 6 月于北京

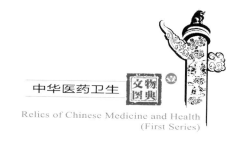

目　录

第二章 清 代

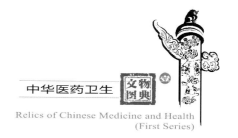

中华医药卫生

Relics of Chinese Medicine and Health
(First Series)

Contents

Chapter Two   Qing Dynasty

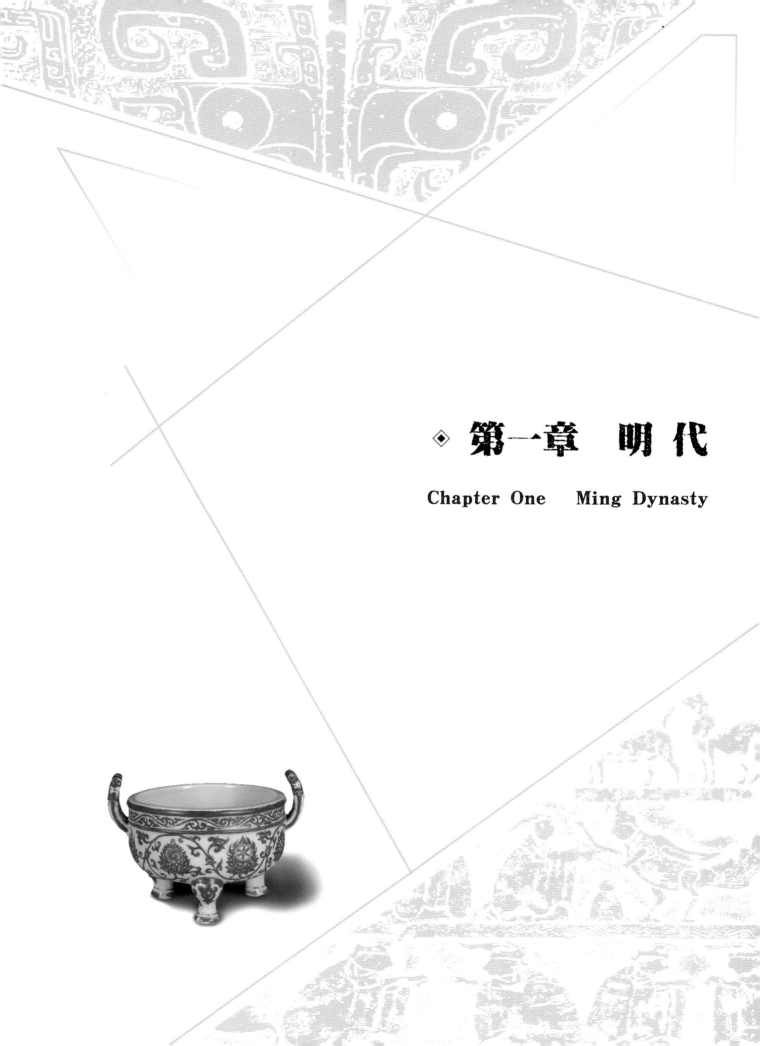

◈ 第一章 明 代

Chapter One　Ming Dynasty

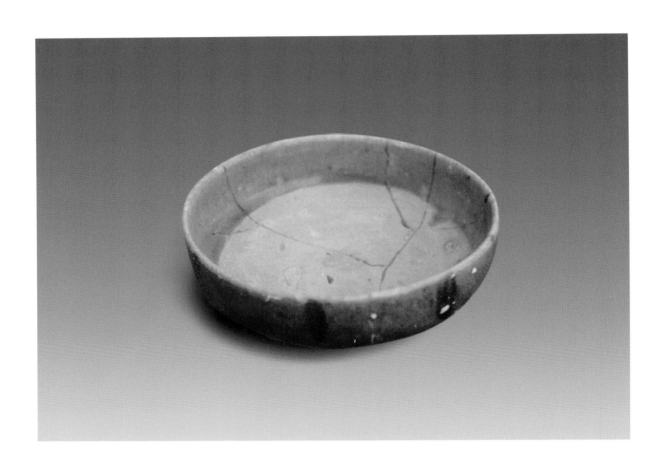

龙泉窑擂钵

明

瓷质

口外径 14.9 厘米，底径 8.9 厘米，通高 5.28 厘米，重 397.5 克

Mortar of Longquan Kiln

Ming Dynasty

Porcelain

Mouth Outer Diameter 14.9 cm/ Bottom Diameter 8.9 cm/ Height 5.28 cm/ Weight 397.5 g

形似盘，直口，平底。通体施青釉。用于研
细药物。

广东中医药博物馆藏

The mortar is shaped like a plate with a vertical
mouth and a flat bottom. The whole body is
covered with blue-and-white glaze. The mortar
was used for porphyrizing drug ingredients.
Preserved in Guangdong Chinese Medicine Museum

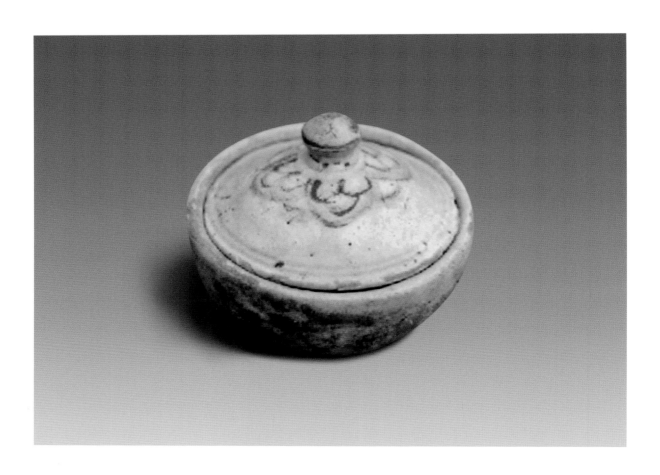

龙泉窑瓷钵

明

瓷质

口外径 7.5 厘米，底径 4 厘米，通高 3.3 厘米，带盖高 6.2 厘米，深 3 厘米，重 143 克

Porcelain Mortar of Longquan Kiln

Ming Dynasty

Porcelain

Mouth Outer Diameter 7.5 cm/ Bottom Diameter 4 cm/ Height 3.3 cm/ Height With Lid 6.2 cm/ Depth 3 cm/ Weight 143 g

形似碗，敛口，平底，带盖，盖顶宝珠纽。
用于研细药物。

广东中医药博物馆藏

The mortar is shaped like a bowl with a contracted
mouth, a flat bottom, and a lid. The top of the lid
is covered with a pearl-shaped knob. The mortar
was used for porphyrizing drug ingredients.
Preserved in Guangdong Chinese Medicine Museum

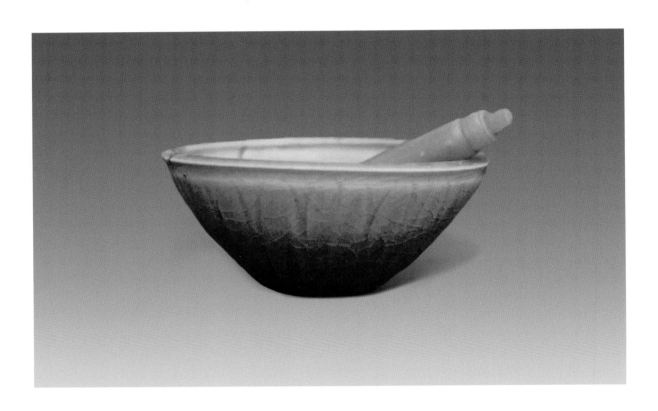

龙泉窑擂钵及杵

明

瓷质

杵：长 13.9 厘米，直径 2.14 厘米，重 120 克

擂钵：口外径 15.26 厘米，底径 5.05 厘米，高 8.23 厘米，深 5.5 厘米，重 535 克

Mortar and Pestle of Longquan Kiln

Ming Dynasty

Porcelain

Pestle: Length 13.9 cm/ Diameter 2.14 cm/ Weight 120 g

Mortar: Mouth Outer Diameter 15.26 cm/ Bottom Diameter 5.05 cm/ Height 8.23 cm/ Depth 5.5 cm/ Weight 535 g

杵为青色玉质，呈棒状，首端呈半球形，尾端有纽。钵为瓷质，敞口，平底。通体施青釉。用于研细药物。

广东中医药博物馆藏

The pestle, made of sapphire, is shaped like a stick. The head of the pestle is hemispherical and its tail has a knob. The mortar, made of porcelain, has a flared mouth and a flat bottom. The whole body of the mortar is covered with green glaze. The collection was used for porphyrizing drug ingredients.

Preserved in Guangdong Chinese Medicine Museum

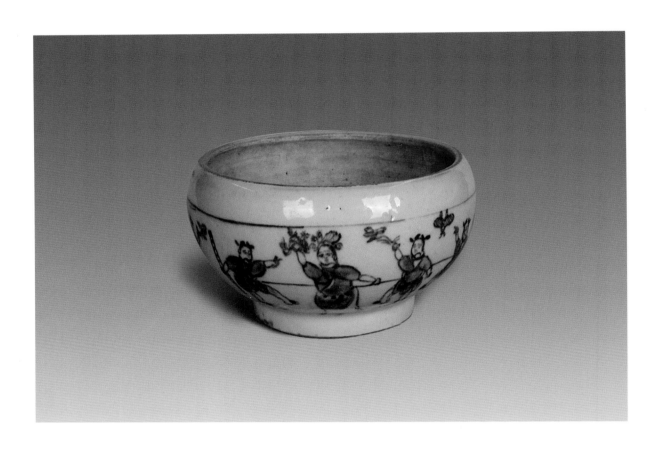

青花研钵

明

瓷质

口内径 12.1 厘米，口外径 13.35 厘米，腹径 14.45 厘米，底径 8.4 厘米，通高 8.1 厘米

Blue-and-white Mortar

Ming Dynasty

Porcelain

Mouth Inner Diameter 12.1 cm/ Mouth Outer Diameter 13.35 cm/ Belly Diameter 14.45 cm/ Bottom Diameter 8.4 cm/ Height 8.1 cm

敛口，平底，圈足。表面绘青花人物故事图，内面及底均无釉。钵内旋纹明显，有使用痕迹。钵底无款识。用于研细药物。1959 年入藏。保存基本完好。

中华医学会 / 上海中医药大学医史博物馆藏

The mortar has a contracted mouth, a flat bottom, and a ring foot. The surface of the mortar is painted with blue-and-white figures. There is no glaze on the interior or the bottom of the mortar. The interior wall of the mortar has spiral patterns and there are traces of using. There is no inscription on the bottom of the mortar. The mortar was used for porphyrizing drug ingredients. It was collected in 1959 and is basically in good condition.

Preserved in Chinese Medical Association/ Museum of Chinese Medicine, Shanghai University of Traditional Chinese Medicine

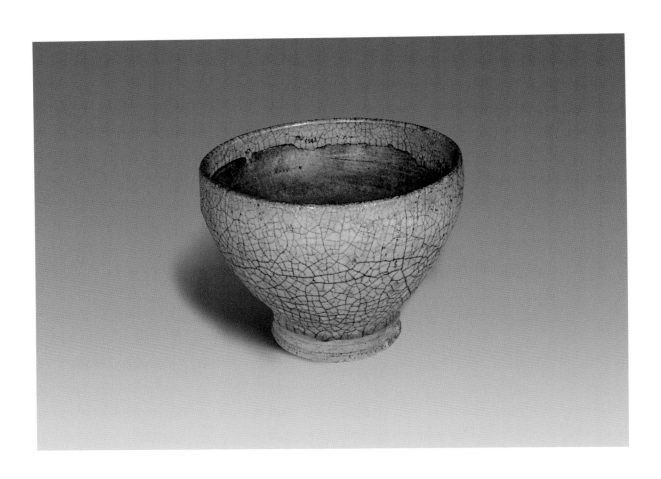

研钵

明

瓷质

口内径 18.2 厘米，口外径 19.2 厘米，腹径 20 厘米，通高 12.2 厘米

Mortar

Ming Dynasty

Porcelain

Mouth Inner Diameter 18.2 cm/ Mouth Outer Diameter 19.2 cm/ Belly Diameter 20 cm/ Height 12.2 cm

形似圆钵，直口微敛，平底，圈足。口沿及
外部施灰绿釉，小开片，钵内及底均无釉。
用于研细药物。1956年入藏。保存基本完好。

中华医学会 / 上海中医药大学医史博物馆藏

The mortar is shaped like a round pot. It has
a straight and slightly contracted mouth, a flat
bottom, and a ring foot. The rim and exterior
wall of the mortar with small cracks are painted
with grayish green glaze. There is no glaze on
the interior wall or on the bottom. The mortar
was used for porphyrizing drug ingredients.
It was collected in the museum in 1956 and is
basically in good condition.
Preserved in Chinese Medical Association/
Museum of Chinese Medicine, Shanghai
University of Traditional Chinese Medicine

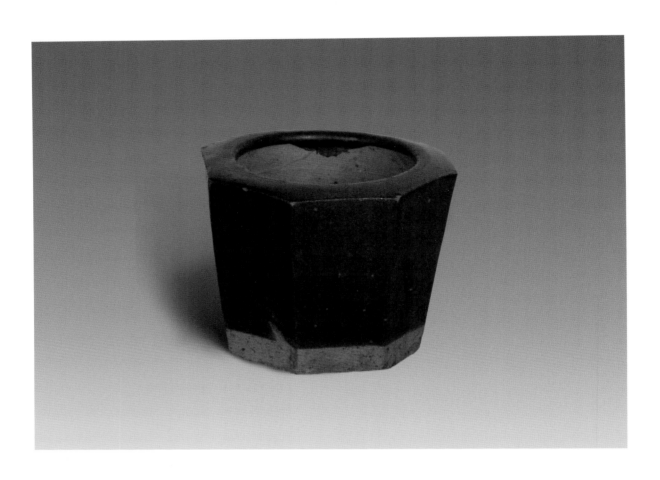

研钵

明

瓷质

宽 12.4 厘米，通高 8.6 厘米

Mortar

Ming Dynasty

Porcelain

Width 12.4 cm/ Height 8.6 cm

八面盆形，敞口，平底。通身施酱色釉，底无釉无款。制药工具，用于研细药物。1959 年入藏。保存基本完好。

中华医学会／上海中医药大学医史博物馆藏

The mortar, which is shaped like an eight-sided basin, has a flared mouth and a flat bottom. The body of the mortar is covered with caramel glaze. There is no inscription or glaze on the bottom. The mortar was used for porphyrizing drug ingredients. It was collected in the museum in 1959 and is basically in good condition. Preserved in Chinese Medical Association/ Museum of Chinese Medicine, Shanghai University of Traditional Chinese Medicine

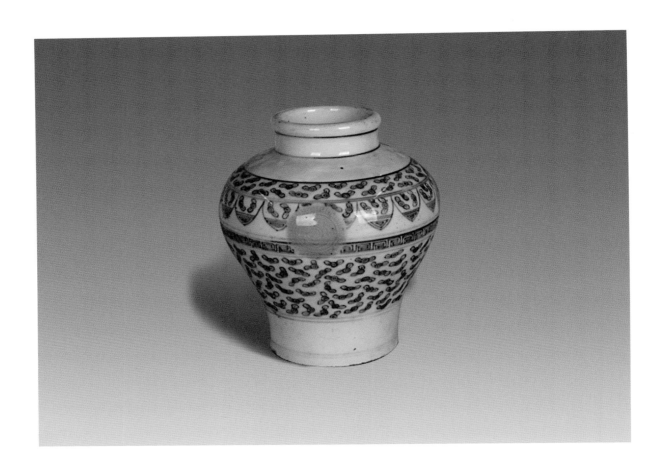

药坛

明

瓷质

口径 4.85 厘米，腹径 9.85 厘米，通高 11.4 厘米

Medicine Jar

Ming Dynasty

Porcelain

Mouth Diameter 4.85 cm/ Belly Diameter 9.85 cm/ Height 11.4 cm

直口略翻沿，平底，圈足。青花釉，绘花草
图案，底有"大明成化年制"款识。用于盛
装细药。1956 年入藏。保存基本完好。

中华医学会 / 上海中医药大学医史博物馆藏

The jar has a vertical mouth with slightly
flared rim, a flat bottom, and a ring foot. The
jar is covered with blue-and-white glaze and
painted with flower and grass patterns. Its
bottom is inscribed with six Chinese characters
reading "Da Ming Cheng Hua Nian Zhi" (made
in Chenghua Period of the Ming Dynasty).
The mortar was used for storing medicine. It
was collected in the museum in 1956 and is
basically in good condition.
Preserved in Chinese Medical Association/
Museum of Chinese Medicine, Shanghai
University of Traditional Chinese Medicine

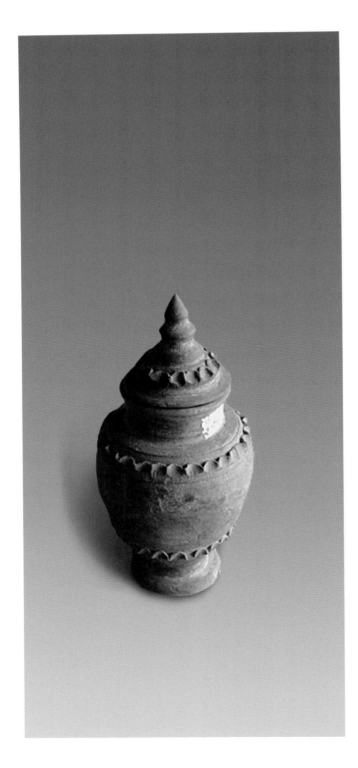

谷仓罐

明

陶质

口径 38 厘米，底径 8 厘米，高 26 厘米

Granary Jar

Ming Dynasty

Pottery

Mouth Diameter 38 cm/ Bottom Diameter 8 cm/

Height 26 cm

器身呈塔形，饼形足。由成都市考古队调拔。

成都中医药大学中医药传统文化博物馆藏

The pottery jar resembles a tower with a cake-shaped foot. It was allocated from Chengdu Archaeological Team.

Preserved in Museum of Traditional Chinese Medicine Culture, Chengdu University of Traditional Chinese Medicine

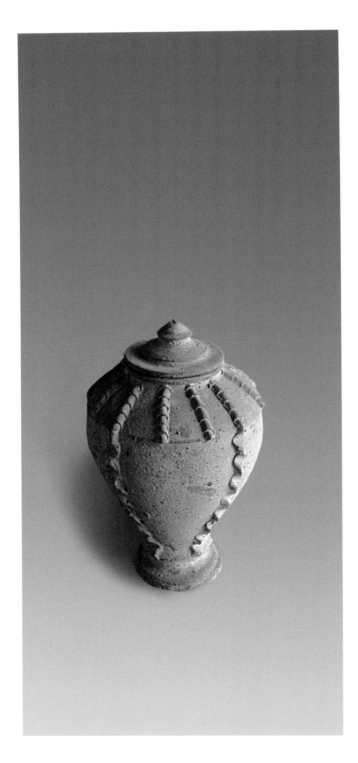

谷仓罐

明

陶质

口径 8 厘米，底径 9 厘米，高 25 厘米

Granary Jar

Ming Dynasty

Pottery

Mouth Diameter 8 cm/ Bottom Diameter 9 cm/

Height 25 cm

鼓肩，腹内收，饼形足，塔形盖，堆塑装饰。
该藏品又称魂瓶，在墓葬中用于镇墓之用，
造型各异。由成都市考古队调拔。

成都中医药大学中医药传统文化博物馆藏

The pottery jar has a bulged shoulder, a tapered belly, a cake-shaped foot, and a tower-shaped lid. The body is decorated with patterns. This collection, also known as soul jar, came in various shapes and was utilized for guarding tombs. The jar was allocated from Chengdu Archaeological Team.

Preserved in Museum of Traditional Chinese Medicine Culture, Chengdu University of Traditional Chinese Medicine

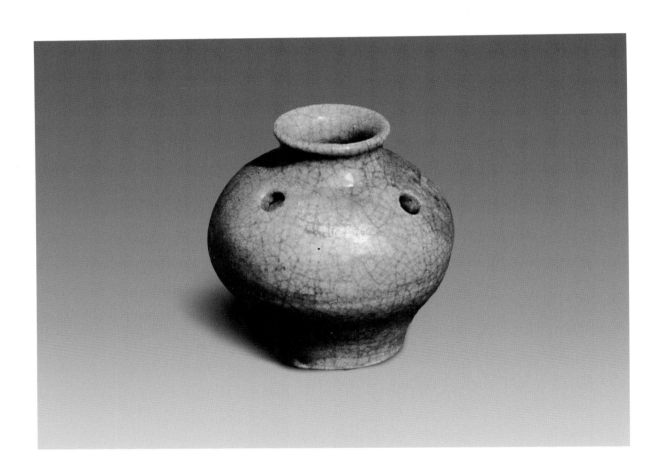

熏罐

明

瓷质

腹径 8.2 厘米，高 8.3 厘米

Incense Pot

Ming Dynasty

Porcelain

Belly Diameter 8.2 cm/ Height 8.3 cm

罐形，无盖。在罐肩上有对称的圆眼四个，罐内盛小斗放置药物，使蒸气从罐口和罐肩四个圆眼中排出，以熏治各类疾病。江苏江阴夏颧墓出土。

江阴博物馆藏

The porcelain pot has no lid. There are four symmetrical round holes on the shoulder. Inside the pot is a dipper for holding medicine. The device can expel steam from the pot mouth and the four holes to treat diseases by smoking. The pot was unearthed from Xia Quan's tomb in Jiangyin City, Jiangsu Province.

Preserved in Jiangyin Museum

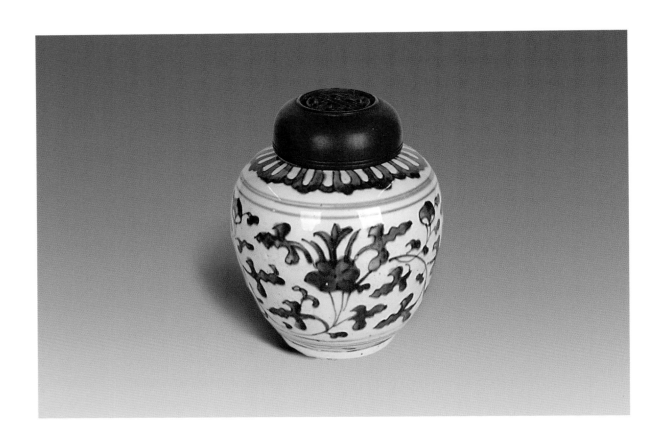

青花瓷药罐

明

瓷质

口内径 6.2 厘米，口外径 7.3 厘米，腹径 15.4 厘米，底径 9.5 厘米，通高 16.3 厘米

Blue-and-white Porcelain Medicine Pot

Ming Dynasty

Porcelain

Mouth Inner Diameter 6.2 cm/ Mouth Outer Diameter 7.3 cm/ Belly Diameter 15.4 cm/ Bottom Diameter 9.5 cm/ Height 16.3 cm

圆罐形，鼓腹，平底，圈足，配红木盖（上有雕刻）。青花瓷，器表绘花卉缠枝图案，底无款识。用于盛装细药。1958 年入藏。保存基本完好。

中华医学会 / 上海中医药大学医史博物馆藏

The round pot, which is made of blue-and-white porcelain, has a bulged belly, a flat bottom, and a ring foot. It has a rosewood lid with engraved patterns on top. The surface of the pot is painted with intertwining branch patterns. There is no inscription on the bottom. The pot was used for storing medicine. It was collected in the museum in 1958 and is basically in good condition.

Preserved in Chinese Medical Association/ Museum of Chinese Medicine, Shanghai University of Traditional Chinese Medicine

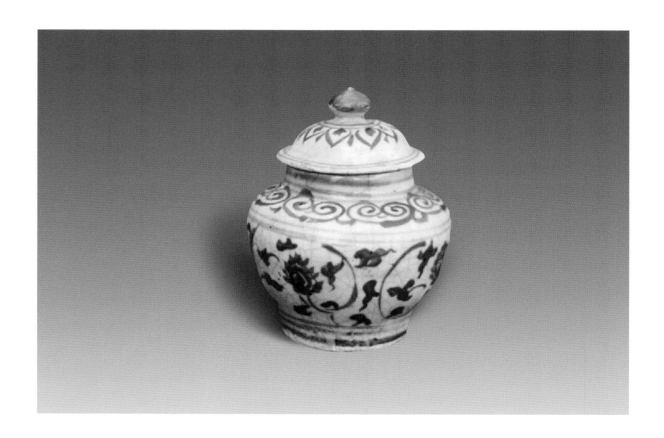

瓷罐

明

瓷质

口外径 5.25 厘米，腹径 9.9 厘米，底径 6 厘米，通高 13.4 厘米，腹深 9.6 厘米，重 329 克

Porcelain Medicine Pot

Ming Dynasty

Porcelain

Mouth Outer Diameter 5.25cm/ Belly Diameter 9.9 cm/ Bottom Diameter 6 cm/ Height 13.4 cm/ Depth 9.6 cm/
Weight 329 g

直口，平肩，圆腹，上鼓下敛，圈足，带盖，
盖顶宝珠纽。器表绘青花花卉图案。用于
盛装细药。

广东中医药博物馆藏

The pot has a vertical mouth, a flat shoulder, a
bulged and tapered belly, and a ring foot. It has
a lid with a pearl-shaped knob. The surface of
the pot is painted with blue-and-white flower
patterns. The pot was used for storing medicine.
Preserved in Guangdong Chinese Medicine Museum

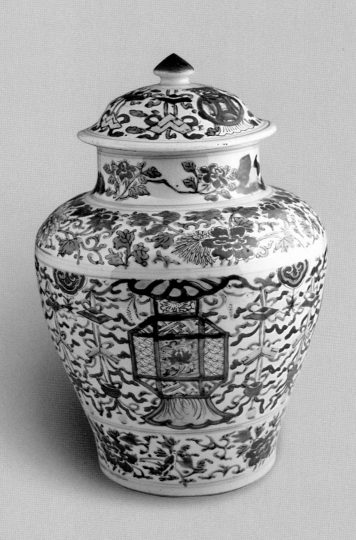

五彩药罐

明

瓷质

上口径 16 厘米，底径 16 厘米

直口，丰肩，斜腹，平底，配有宝珠纽盖。通体施五彩纹饰，色彩鲜艳。御生堂盛装药品器皿。

北京御生堂中医药博物馆藏

Multi-colored Medicine Pot

Qing Dynasty

Porcelain

Upper Mouth Diameter 16 cm/ Bottom Diameter 16 cm

It has a vertical mouth, a plump shoulder, an inclined belly, a flat bottom and a jewelry-shaped knob. Its surface is painted with bright multi-colored patterns. The pot was used for storing medicine in Yu Sheng Tang Drugstore.

Preserved in Chinese Medicine Museum of Beijing Yu Sheng Tang Drugstore

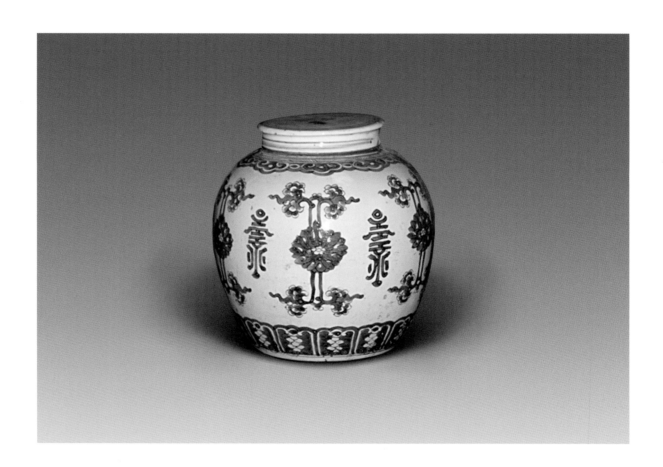

青花药罐

明

瓷质

口径 9 厘米，底径 13.5 厘米，通高 22 厘米，重 2400 克

Blue-and-white Medicine Pot

Ming Dynasty

Porcelain

Mouth Diameter 9 cm/ Bottom Diameter 13.5 cm/ Height 22 cm/ Weight 2,400 g

子母口，圆腹，圈足。器表绘青花"寿"字
图案及变形荷花。用于盛装细药。陕西三原
征集。

陕西医史博物馆藏

The pot has a snap-lid, a round belly, and a
ring foot. The surface of the pot is painted with
one blue-and-white character reading "shou"
(longevity) and transformed lotuses. The pot
was used for storing medicine. It was collected
from Sanyuan County, Shaanxi Province.

Preserved in Shaanxi Museum of Medical History

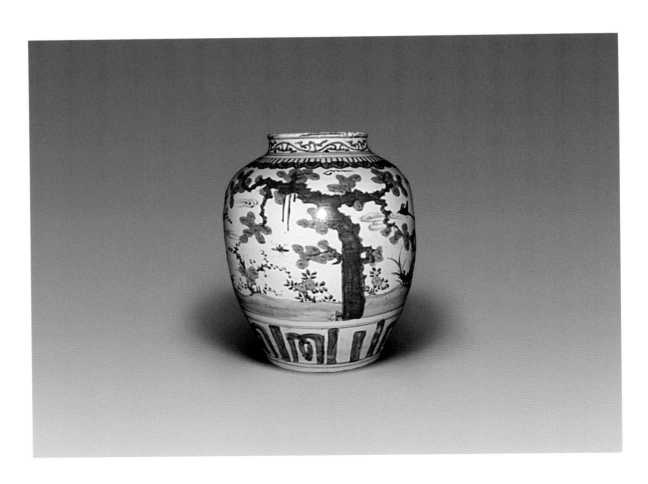

青花药罐

明

瓷质

口径 17.5 厘米，底径 22 厘米，通高 40 厘米，重 9400 克

Blue-and-white Medicine Pot

Ming Dynasty

Porcelain

Mouth Diameter 17.5 cm/ Bottom Diameter 22 cm/ Height 40 cm/ Weight 9,400 g

圆唇，高领，曲腹，圈足，口沿微残。器表绘
青花松竹梅"岁寒三友"图案。用于盛装细药。
1983 年入藏。陕西泾阳万灵堂药店征集。

陕西医史博物馆藏

The pot has a round mouth with slightly damaged
rim, a long neck, a cambered belly, and a ring
foot. The surface of the pot is painted with
patterns of the three durable plants of winter —
pine, bamboo and plum — in blue-and-white
glaze. The pot was used for storing medicine. It
was collected from Wan Ling Tang Drug Store,
Jingyang County, Shaanxi Province, in 1983.
Preserved in Shaanxi Museum of Medical History

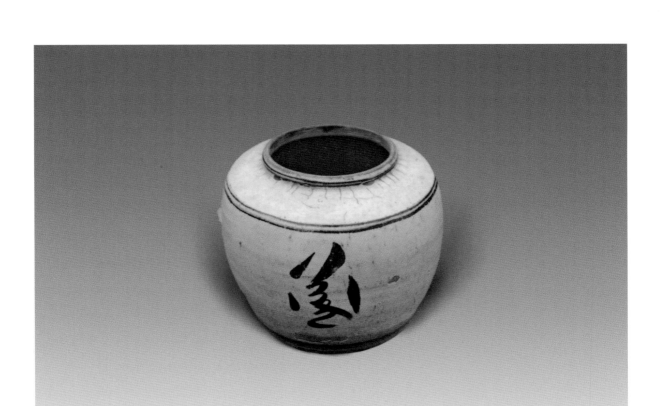

磁州窑瓷罐

明

瓷质

口外径 12.6 厘米，腹径 22.3 厘米，底径 18 厘米，通高 19.7 厘米，腹深 18.4 厘米，重 2500 克

Porcelain Pot of Cizhou Kiln

Ming Dynasty

Porcelain

Mouth Outer Diameter 12.6 cm/ Belly Diameter 22.3 cm/ Bottom Diameter 18 cm/ Height 19.7 cm/ Belly Depth 18.4 cm/ Weight 2,500 g

直口，鼓腹，平底。通体施白釉，腹部书写
酱色文字。用于盛物。

广东中医药博物馆藏

The porcelain pot has a vertical mouth, a bulged
belly and a flat bottom. Its body is coated with
white glaze and its belly is inscribed with brown
Chinese characters. The pot was utilized as a
container.

Preserved in Guangdong Chinese Medicine Museum

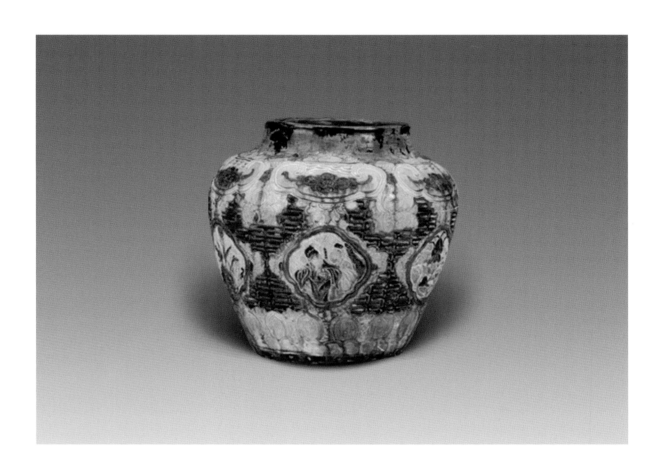

珐花镂空罐

明

陶质

口径 21.5 厘米，高 34.5 厘米

Hollowed Pot with Contour-raised Design

Ming Dynasty

Pottery

Mouth Diameter 21.5 cm/ Height 34.5 cm

罐为陶胎，大口，宽肩，平底。罐腹部胎体
为内、外两层，内层为光素无釉的涩胎，外
层施以深蓝色衬底的珐花釉。

山西博物院藏

The pottery pot has a big mouth, a broad
shoulder and a flat bottom. Its inner body is
coated with no glaze while the outer body is
coated with dark blue contour-raised design
glaze.

Preserved in Shanxi Museum

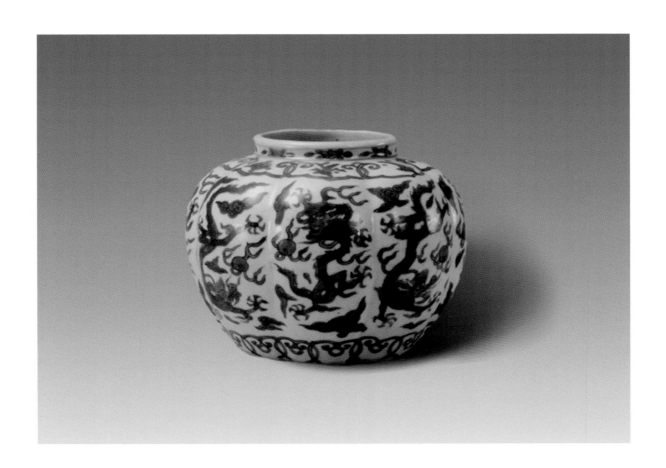

青花云龙纹瓜棱罐

明

瓷质

口径 7.8 厘米，底径 9.5 厘米，高 12.3 厘米

Blue-and-white Pot with Dragon among Clouds Patterns

Ming Dynasty

Porcelain

Mouth Diameter 7.8 cm/ Bottom Diameter 9.5 cm/ Height 12.3 cm

直口，短颈，腹部呈瓜棱形，平底，圈足。胎细色白，釉色白中闪青。八道瓜棱上各绘青花云龙纹，龙首方向交错排列。龙首向上者圆目张口，怒发前冲；龙首向下者翘首舞爪，龙的首尾处绘有朵云与火珠。器底青花楷书"大明万历年制"。景德镇窑瓷罐瓜棱上绘制青花龙纹，实属罕见。

德州市文化局藏

This pot has a vertical mouth, a short neck, a melon-shaped belly, a flat bottom and a ring foot. The pottery body is white and fine and the glaze is white mixed with blue. The eight melon bulges are decorated with blue-and-white dragon among clouds whose heads are intersecting with each other. The dragons that hold their heads up are opening their mouth with staring eyes and the dragons that lower their heads are waving their claws. There are cloud and fire pearl patterns around the dragons' heads and tails. The bottom of the pot is inscribed in regular script with six Chinese characters reading "Da Ming Wan Li Nian Zhi" (made during Wanli Period of the Ming Dynasty). It was very rare to have dragon patterns painted on the bulges of blue-and-white porcelain pots of Jingdezhen Kiln.

Preserved in Dezhou Municipal Bureau of Culture

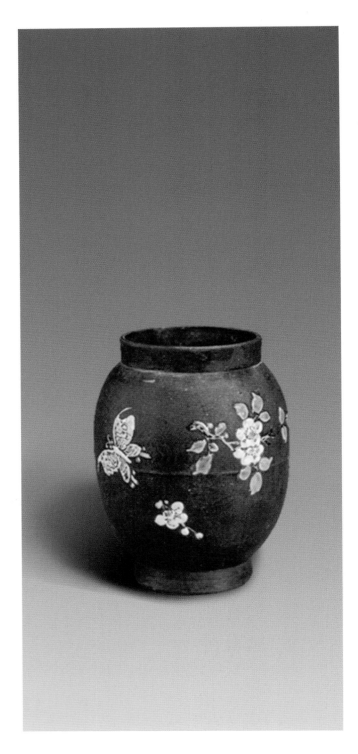

翻瓷花鸟纹罐

明

瓷质

口径 7.4 厘米，高 14.2 厘米

侈口，溜肩，深腹。口、底大小相当，腹径
略鼓于口、底。罐内外无釉，只刷浆水，赭色。
腹部饰白色喜鹊、蝴蝶、折枝梅花等图案。

山西博物院藏

Porcelain Pot with Flower and Bird Patterns

Ming Dynasty

Porcelain

Mouth Diameter 7.4 cm/ Height 14.2 cm

This pot has a wide flared mouth, a narrow and
sloping shoulder, and a deep belly which is slight
wider than the mouth and the bottom. The interior
and exterior are not covered with glaze but only
ocherous seriflux. The belly is decorated with
white magpies, butterflies and plucked plums.

Preserved in Shanxi Museum

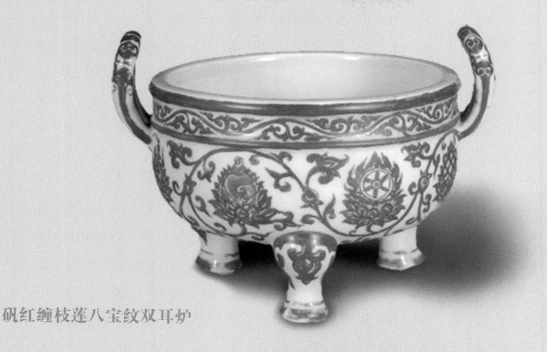

矾红缠枝莲八宝纹双耳炉

明

瓷质

口径 14.3 厘米，高 10.4 厘米

直口，厚唇，上腹较直，下腹微鼓，圜底，蹄形三足，腹部伸出的两附耳均向内弓。胎洁白细腻，釉色白而润泽。器表通体用矾红描绘纹饰。口沿饰卷草纹一周，腹部饰缠枝莲纹，莲朵上衬以轮、螺、伞、幢、花、瓶、鱼、结八宝，耳与足根部绘垂云纹。

河北博物院藏

Two-eared Censer with Patterns of Lotuses and Eight Treasures

Ming Dynasty

Porcelain

Mouth Diameter 14.3 cm/ Height 10.4 cm

The porcelain censer has a vertical mouth, a thick lip, a belly vertical in the upper part and bulged in the lower part, a round bottom, and three hook-shaped feet. A pair of handle extending from the belly turn inside. The body base is white and fine and the glaze is white, smooth and mellow. The surface of the body is painted iron red. Its mouth rim is decorated with a circle of scroll designs. The belly is patterned with intertwining lotuses on which there are eight treasures including wheel, whorl, umbrella, pennant, flower, vase, fish, and knot. On its ears and feet are descending cloud patterns.

Preserved in Hebei Museum

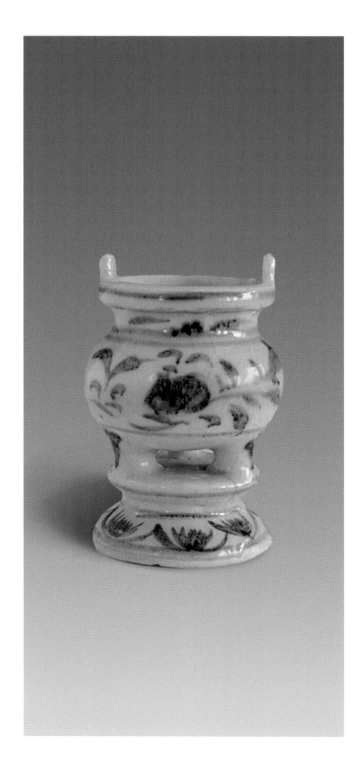

青花缠枝莲花三足双耳炉

明

瓷质

口径 5.3 厘米，高 9.3 厘米

Blue-and-white Censer with Intertwining Lotuses, Three Feet and Two Ears

Ming Dynasty

Porcelain

Mouth Diameter 5.3 cm/ Height 9.3 cm

洗口，短颈，丰腹，腹下置三鬲式足，下乘
一圆形座。口唇设鋬式对称耳。全身满施白
釉，口缘有缩釉处闪淡淡的火石红色。腹绘
缠枝莲纹，口缘绘两条弦纹，颈部绘回纹。
青花呈色浓而略灰，应是国产料。为明初期
作品。

周振武藏

The porcelain censer has a shallow mouth, a
short neck, a swelling belly, three feet like a
Li pot, a round base, and a pair of symmetrical
ears on its mouth. The whole body is coated
with white glaze. There are intertwining lotuses
around its belly, two bow string patterns on
its mouth rim, and fret patterns on its neck. Its
material should be domestic cobalt as the blue
is heavy and slightly gray. The censer dates
back to the Early Ming Dynasty.

Collected by Zhou Zhenwu

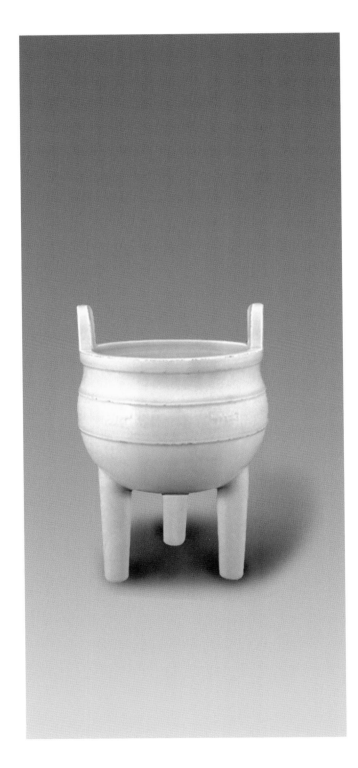

德化窑弦纹双耳三足炉

明

瓷质

口径 18 厘米，高 27 厘米，足距 14 厘米

Censer with Bow String Patterns, Three Feet and Two Ears, Dehua Kiln

Ming Dynasty

Porcelain

Mouth Diameter 18 cm/ Height 27 cm/

Distance Between Feet 14 cm

炉体厚唇圆腹，下承三柱足，口上立对称冲
天耳，腹部凸起双弦纹，弦纹之间锦地仿古
铜纹饰。1987 年美籍华人、医学博士蔡流轮
捐赠。

　　　　　　　　故宫博物院藏

The porcelain censer has a thick lip, a round
belly, three feet, a pair of ears standing skyward
on its mouth, and two bulged bow string
patterns on the belly. Between the bow string
patterns there are bronze-like decorations. The
censer was donated by Chinese-American Mr.
Cai Liulun, M.D., in 1987.

Preserved in The Palace Museum

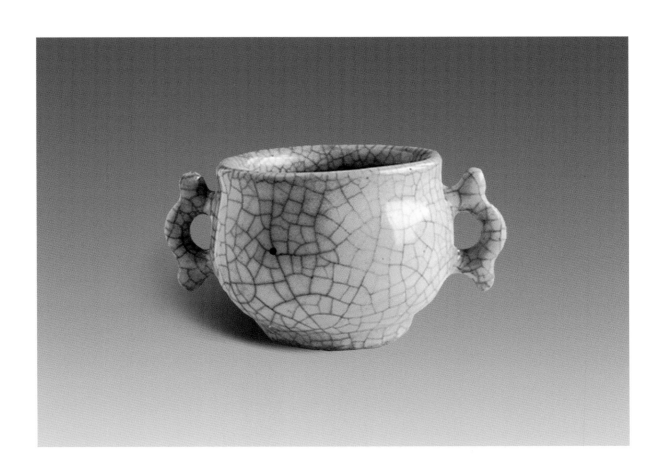

哥窑釉双耳炉

明

瓷质

口径 7.8 厘米，高 6.5 厘米

Glazed Censer with Two Ears, Ge Kiln

Ming Dynasty

Porcelain

Mouth Diameter 7.8 cm/ Height 6.5 cm

侈口，鼓腹，平底，圈足，双如意形耳。釉厚莹润，开红色纹片。

章兆泉藏

The porcelain censer has an everted mouth, a bulged belly, a flat bottom, a ring foot, and a pair of ears shaped like Ruyi,a traditional propitions decoration. The glaze is mellow and smooth with red crackles.

Collected by Zhang Zhaoquan

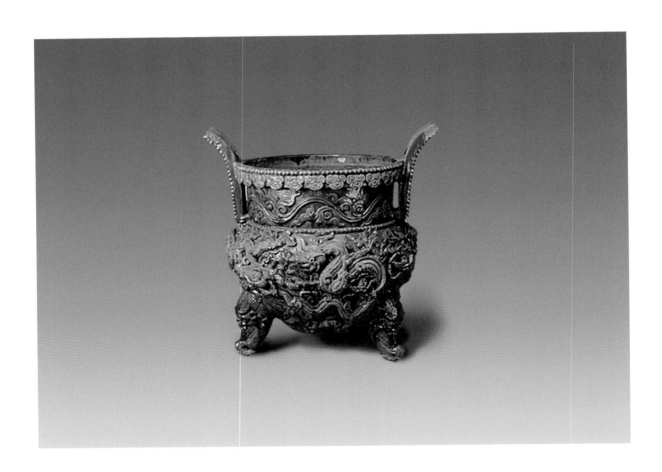

黄绿釉蟠龙大炉

明

陶质

口径 53 厘米，高 73 厘米

Yellowish Green-glazed Censer with Coiled Dragons

Ming Dynasty

Pottery

Mouth Diameter 53 cm/ Height 73 cm

鼎式炉，夹砂陶胎，平沿，直颈，鼓腹，圜底。肩两侧有长方形双耳，耳外撇，螭头形足。通体施黄绿色釉，口沿及双耳饰连珠纹，口沿下垂如意纹，颈部饰卷草纹，腹部为龙戏牡丹花。此炉胎体厚重，釉色深沉，形象庄严。

山西博物院藏

The censer is shaped like a Ding-vessel, with a sand-pottery body , a flat rim, a vertical neck, a bulged belly, and a round bottom. On both sides of the shoulder a pair of rectangular handles extend out. The feet resemble the head of a Chi dragon. The whole body of the censer is covered with yellowish green glaze. There are pearl patterns on its mouth rim and ears, Ruyi patterns on the under part of its rim, scroll designs on its neck, and dragons playing with peonies on its belly. The material is thick and heavy while the glaze is dark, showing dignity.
Preserved in Shanxi Museum

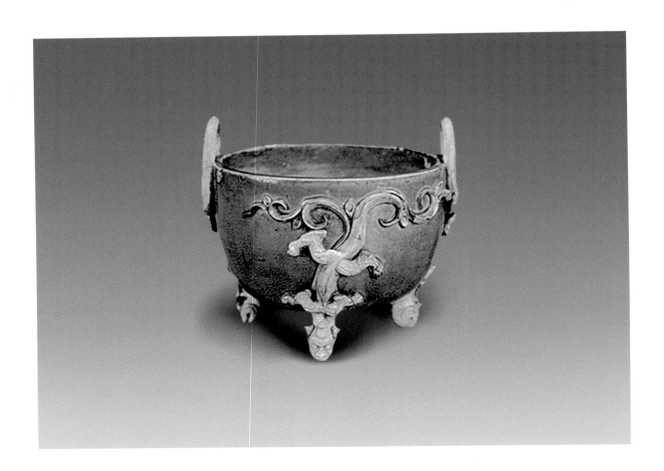

孔雀绿釉蟠螭炉

明

瓷质

口径 20 厘米，高 19.2 厘米

Peacock-green Glazed Censer with Panchi Dragons

Ming Dynasty

Porcelain

Mouth Diameter 20 cm/ Height 19.2 cm

直口，平沿，圆腹，圜底。通体施孔雀绿釉，釉层较薄，有细小开片，器面上堆塑三只倒体蟠螭贯穿整个炉身，螭首作炉足，螭身为白色，倒爬于炉壁，螭尾弯作炉耳。

山西博物院藏

The porcelain censer has a vertical mouth, a flat rim, a bulged belly, and round bottom. The whole body is covered with peacock-green glaze, which is thin with fine crackles. Three inverted Panchi dragons surround the surface of the censer, their heads serving as the censer's feet, their inverted white bodies climbing the wall, and their tails serving as the censer's ears.

Preserved in Shanxi Museum

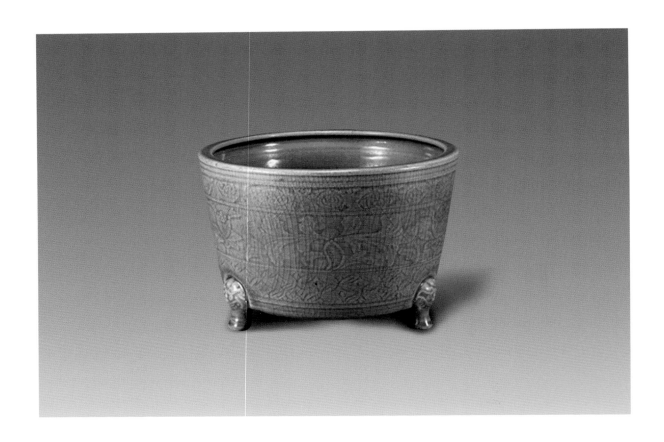

龙泉窑暗花折枝花卉纹筒式三足炉

明

瓷质

口径 25.8 厘米，底径 11 厘米，高 16.9 厘米

Cylinder-shaped Censer with Plucked Flower Patterns and Three Feet, Longquan Kiln

Ming Dynasty

Porcelain

Mouth Diameter 25.8 cm/ Bottom Diameter 11 cm/ Height 16.9 cm

炉呈筒状，腹向下渐收，下承三个印兽头的
蹄形足。青绿色釉，釉质清亮透明，开细片纹，
底部露胎微外凸，见大片火石红，胎体厚重。
腹部刻云头纹和折枝牡丹纹。

常州博物馆藏

The cylinder-shaped censer has a tapered belly
and three hook-shaped feet with animal heads.
The whole body is coated with green glaze,
which is clear and bright with fine crackles. The
slightly convex bottom is exposed with no glaze
but a large part of kiln red. The pottery body
is thick and heavy.Its belly is decorated with
patterns of clouds and plucked peonies.
Preserved in Changzhou Museum

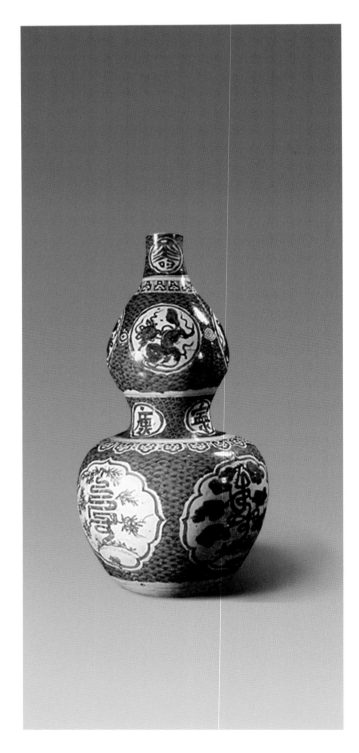

"福寿康宁"青花葫芦药瓶

明

瓷质

口径 5.5 厘米，底径 14.5 厘米，高 50.5 厘米

Blue-and-white Gourd-shaped Medicine Bottle with Auspicious Words

Ming Dynasty

Porcelain

Mouth Diameter 5.5 cm/ Bottom Diameter 14.5 cm/ Height 50.5 cm

葫芦形，小直口，束腰，鼓腹，平底。为青
花瓷，上部绘以狮子戏球，灵飞生动；中部
以花枝组成"福寿康宁"四字；下部绘有松、
柏、梅等图案，取意吉祥。用于装药。

上海中医药博物馆藏

The bottle, which is shaped like a gourd, has a small vertical mouth, a narrow waist, a bulged belly, and a flat bottom. It is made of blue-and-white porcelain. The upper part of the bottle is painted with lions playing with balls. The middle part of the bottle is decorated with four characters reading "Fu Shou Kang Ning" (good fortune, long life, good health, and peacefulness) in flower branches. The lower part of the bottle is painted with pine, cypress and plum patterns which carry auspicious meanings. It was used for storing medicine. Preserved in Shanghai Museum of Traditional Chinese Medicine

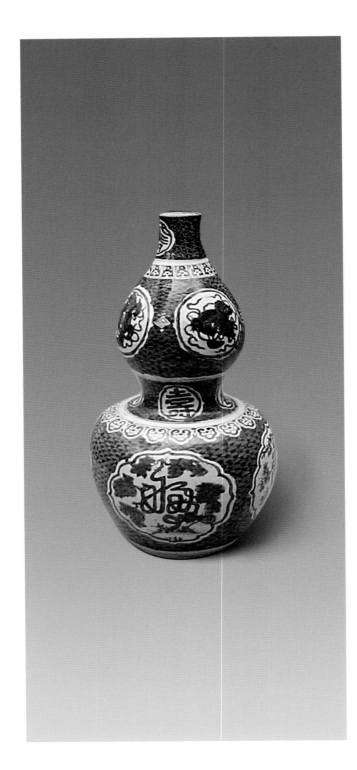

葫芦药瓶

明

瓷质

口外径 5.4 厘米，上腹径 17.5 厘米，下腹径
26.5 厘米，底径 14 厘米，通高 49.3 厘米

Gourd-shaped Medicine Bottle

Ming Dynasty

Porcelain

Mouth Outer Diameter 5.4 cm/ Upper Belly
Diameter 17.5 cm/ Lower Belly Diameter 26.5 cm/
Bottom Diameter 14 cm/ Height 49.3 cm

葫芦形，小直口，束腰，鼓腹，平底。为青花瓷，沿口书篆体"寿"字，上部有狮子戏球图，腰部正楷"福寿康宁"，下部绘松、柏、梅图案。用于装药。1954 年入藏。保存基本完好。

中华医学会 / 上海中医药大学医史博物馆藏

The gourd-shaped bottle has a small vertical mouth, a narrow waist, a bulged belly, and a flat bottom. It is made of blue-and-white porcelain. The edge of the bottle is painted with a seal-script character reading "Shou" (longevity). The waist of the bottle is inscribed with four regular-script words reading "Fu Shou Kang Ning" (good fortune, long life, good health, and peacefulness) in flower branches. The upper part of the bottle is painted with lions playing with balls while the lower part is painted with pine, cypress and plum patterns. The bottle was used for storing medicine. It was collected in the museum in 1954 and is still basically in good condition.

Preserved in Chinese Medical Association/ Museum of Chinese Medicine, Shanghai University of Traditional Chinese Medicine

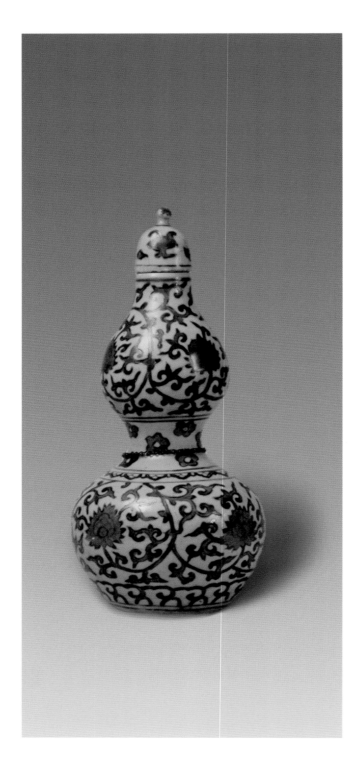

黄釉青花葫芦瓶

明

瓷质

口径 3 厘米，底径 6.5 厘米，通高 23 厘米

Blue-and-white Gourd-shaped Bottle with Yellow Glaze

Ming Dynasty

Porcelain

Mouth Diameter 3 cm/ Bottom Diameter 6.5 cm/

Height 23 cm

葫芦形，圆盖圆纽，子母口，束腰，平底，矮圈足。为青花瓷，通体施黄釉，釉下绘青花缠枝莲花、梅花及蝙蝠。青花色泽浓重，与黄釉相映，显得格外艳丽。底有青花楷书"大明嘉靖年制"款。清乾隆五十二年 (1787) 御赐岱庙作祭器。

泰安市博物馆藏

The gourd-shaped bottle has a round lid, a round button, a snap-lid, a narrow waist, a flat bottom, and a low ring foot. It is made of blue-and-white porcelain. The body of the bottle is covered with yellow glaze. The surface of the bottle is painted with blue-and-white intertwining lotuses, plums and bats under the glaze. The bottom of the bottle is inscribed with six Chinese words in regular script reading "Da Ming Jia Jing Nian Zhi" (made in Jiajing Period of the Ming Dynasty) indicating the year when it was made. The sacrificial vessel was bestowed by the emperor to Dai Temple in the 52nd year of Qianlong Reign (1787) in the Qing Dynasty.

Preserved in Tai'an Museum

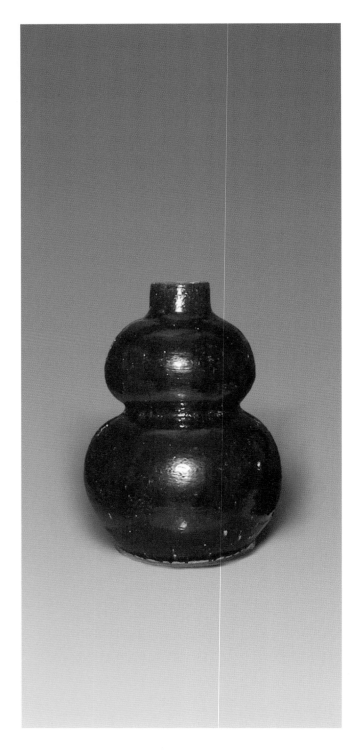

瓷药瓶

明

瓷质

口外径 17.7 厘米，口内径 14.8 厘米，上腹围 143 厘米，下腹围 194 厘米，腰围 112 厘米，通高 96.5 厘米

Porcelain Medicine Pot

Ming Dynasty

Porcelain

Mouth Outer Diameter 17.7 cm/ Mouth Inner Diameter 14.8 cm/ Upper Waistline 143 cm/ Lower Waistline 194 cm/ Waistline 112 cm/ Height 96.5 cm

葫芦形，小直口，束腰，鼓腹，平底。通身
施黑釉，釉面光亮，瓷胎表面凹凸不平整。
用于装药。1960 年入藏。保存基本完好。

中华医学会 / 上海中医药大学医史博物馆藏

The gourd-shaped pot has a small vertical
mouth, a narrow waist, a bulged belly, and a flat
bottom. The surface of the pot is covered with
shiny black glaze. The surface of the porcelain
is not smooth. The pot was used for storing
medicine. It was collected in the museum in
1960 and is basically in good condition.

Preserved in Chinese Medical Association/
Museum of Chinese Medicine, Shanghai
University of Traditional Chinese Medicine

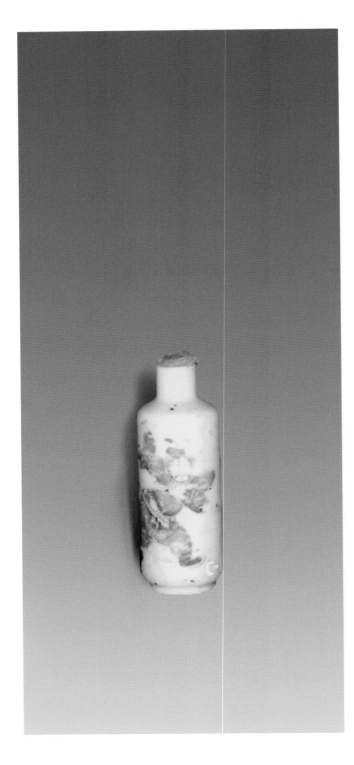

瓷药瓶

明

瓷质

口径 1.1 厘米，底径 2.1 厘米，通高 7 厘米，
重 360 克

Porcelain Medicine Bottle

Ming Dynasty

Porcelain

Mouth Diameter 1.1 cm/ Bottom Diameter 2.1 cm/

Height 7 cm/ Weight 360 g

直口，折肩，直腹，圈足。白釉，红色彩绘
人物图，底有"成化年制"。用于盛装细药。
陕西临潼征集。

陕西医史博物馆藏

The bottle has a vertical mouth, a square
shoulder, a vertical belly, and a ring foot. It is
covered with white glaze and painted with red
figures. The bottom of the bottle is inscribed
with four characters reading "Cheng Hua Nian
Zhi" indicating the year when it was made. The
bottle was used for storing medicine. It was
collected from Lintong District of Xi'an City,
Shaanxi Province.

Preserved in Shaanxi Museum of Medical History

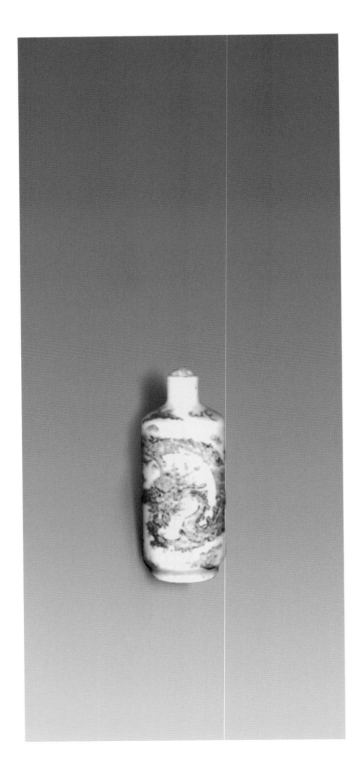

瓷药瓶

明

瓷质

口径 1.1 厘米，底径 2.4 厘米，通高 7 厘米，

重 46.5 克

Porcelain Medicine Bottle

Ming Dynasty

Porcelain

Mouth Diameter 1.1 cm/ Bottom Diameter 2.4 cm/

Height 7 cm/ Weight 46.5 g

直口，折肩，直腹，圈足。白釉，红色彩绘
龙飞舞图。用于盛装细药。陕西临潼征集。

陕西医史博物馆藏

The bottle has a vertical mouth, a square
shoulder, a straight belly, and a ring foot. It is
painted with patterns of red dancing dragons.
The bottle was used for storing medicine. It was
collected from Lintong District of Xi'an City,
Shaanxi Province.

Preserved in Shaanxi Museum of Medical History

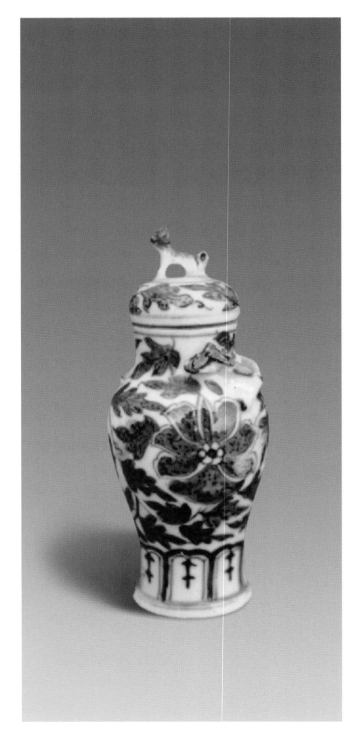

青花药用瓷瓶

明

瓷质

口外径3.8厘米，腹径5.9厘米，底径4.3厘米，

通高 14.2 厘米，腹深 9.5 厘米，重 175 克

Blue-and-white Porcelain Medicine Jar

Ming Dynasty

Porcelain

Mouth Outer Diameter 3.8 cm/ Belly Diameter

5.9 cm/ Bottom Diameter 4.3 cm/ Height 14.2 cm/

Belly Depth 9.5 cm/ Weight 175 g

直口，削肩，鼓腹，其下收敛，平底，盖顶，
一兽形（狗）纽。用于盛装细药。

广东中医药博物馆藏

The jar has a vertical mouth, a sloping shoulder,
a bulged and tapered belly, and a flat bottom. Its
lid has a dog-shaped knob. The jar was used for
storing medicine.

Preserved in Guangdong Chinese Medicine Museum

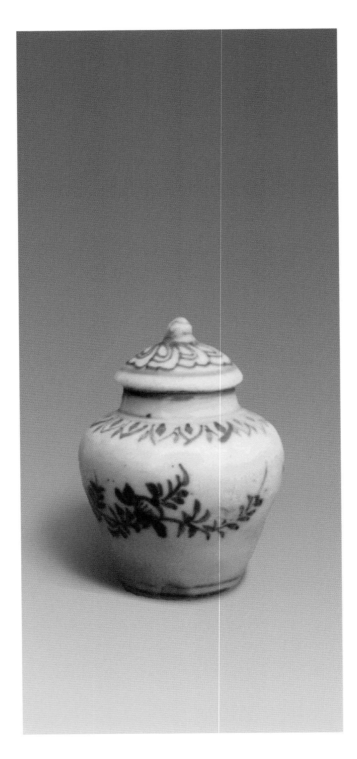

青花药用盖瓶

明

瓷质

口外径3.6厘米，腹径6.7厘米，底径4.1厘米，

通高8.7厘米，腹深6.4厘米，重111克

Blue-and-white Medicine Jar

Ming Dynasty

Porcelain

Mouth Outer Diameter 3.6 cm/ Belly Diameter

6.7 cm/ Bottom Diameter 4.1 cm/ Height 8.7 cm/

Belly Depth 6.4 cm/ Weight 111 g

直口，高领，圆肩，腹部上鼓下敛，平底，带盖，
盖顶圆形纽。用于盛装细药。

广东中医药博物馆藏

The jar has a vertical mouth, a sloping shoulder, a
bulged and tapered belly, and a flat bottom. Its lid
has a round knob. The jar was used for storing
medicine.

Preserved in Guangdong Chinese Medicine Museum

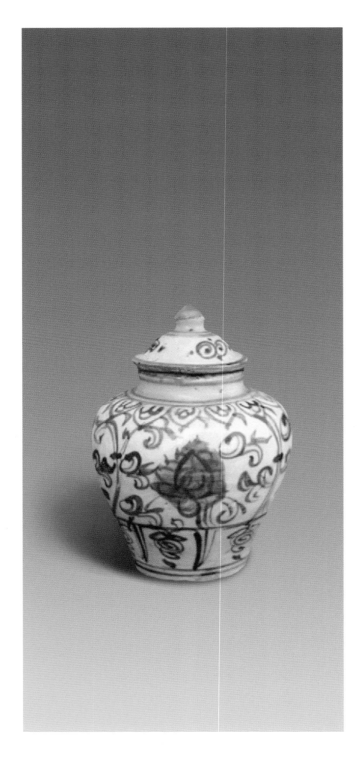

青花药用盖瓶

明

瓷质

口外径6厘米，腹外径10.2厘米，底径6.4厘米，

通高 12.1 厘米，腹深 7.9 厘米，重 320 克

Blue-and-white Medicine Jar

Ming Dynasty

Porcelain

Mouth Outer Diameter 6 cm/ Belly Outer Diameter
10.2 cm/ Bottom Diameter 6.4 cm/ Height 12.1 cm/
Belly Depth 7.9 cm/ Weight 320 g

直口，耸肩，圆腹，上鼓下敛，平底，盖顶
宝珠纽。用于盛装细药。

广东中医药博物馆藏

The jar has a vertical mouth, a shrugged shoulder,
a bulged and tapered belly, and a flat bottom. Its
lid has a pearl-shaped knob. The jar was used
for storing medicine.

Preserved in Guangdong Chinese Medicine Museum

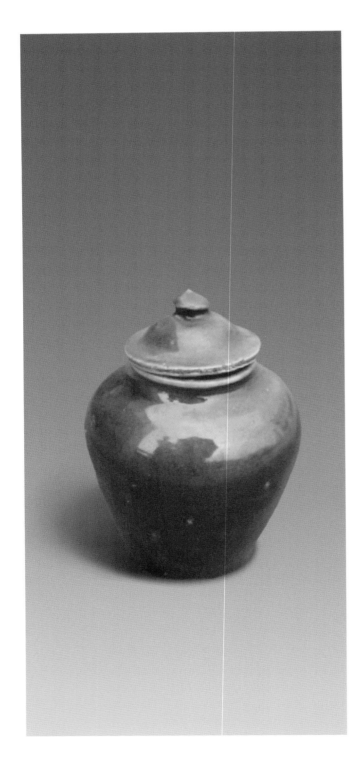

祭蓝药用盖瓶

明

瓷质

口径 4.87 厘米，最大腹径 8.4 厘米，底径 5.8 厘米，通高 13 厘米，腹深 8.9 厘米，重 240 克

Sacrificial Blue Medicine Bottle with Lid

Ming Dynasty

Porcelain

Mouth Diameter 4.87 cm/ Maximum Belly Diameter 8.4 cm/ Bottom Diameter 5.8 cm/ Height 13 cm/ Belly Depth 8.9 cm/ Weight 240 g

侈口，短颈，腹上鼓下敛，平底，带盖，盖
顶宝珠纽与盖形相似。用于盛装细药。

广东中医药博物馆藏

The medicine jar has a wide flared mouth, a
short neck, a bulged and tapered belly, and a flat
bottom. On the top of its lid is a pearl-shaped
knob, which is similar in shape to the lid itself.
The jar was utilized for storing fine medicine.

Preserved in Guangdong Chinese Medicine Museum

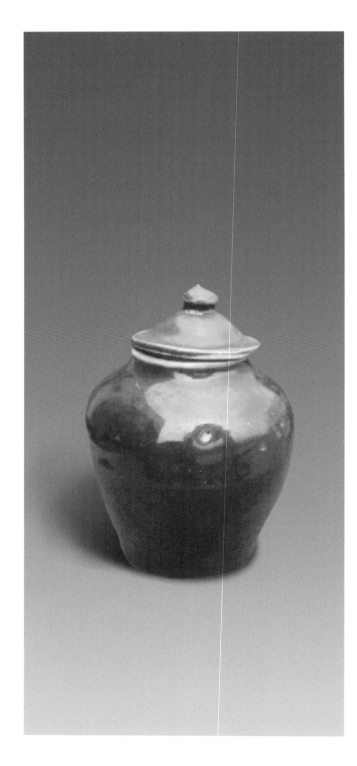

祭蓝药用盖瓶

明

瓷质

口径 4.9 厘米，腹径 8.74 厘米，底径 5.8 厘米，

通高 12 厘米，腹深 8.7 厘米， 重 255 克

Sacrificial Blue Medicine Jar with Lid

Ming Dynasty

Porcelain

Mouth Diameter 4.9 cm/ Belly Diameter 8.74 cm/

Bottom Diameter 5.8 cm/ Height 12 cm/ Belly

Depth 8.7 cm/ Weight 255 g

侈口，短颈，腹上鼓下敛，平底，带盖，盖
顶宝珠纽与盖形相似。用于盛装细药。

广东中医药博物馆藏

The medicine jar, which is made of porcelain,
has a flared mouth, a short neck, a bulged and
tapered belly, and a flat bottom. On the top of
its lid is a pearl-shaped knob, which is similar
in shape to the lid itself. The jar was utilized for
storing fine medicine.

Preserved in Guangdong Chinese Medicine Museum

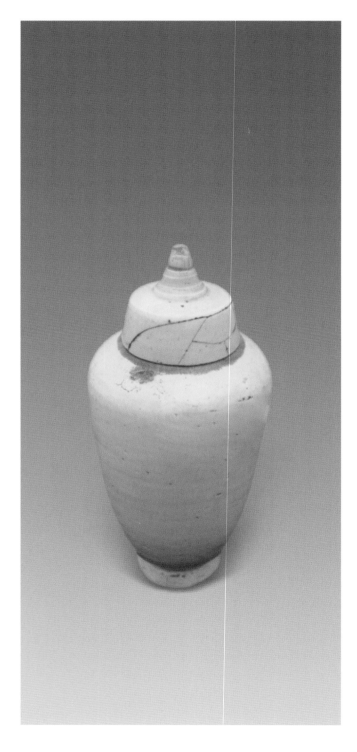

白釉盖瓶

明

瓷质

口外径 7.3 厘米，腹径 15.2 厘米，底径 8 厘米，带盖通高 32.5 厘米，腹深 23.2 厘米，重 2300 克

White-glazed Jar with Lid

Ming Dynasty

Porcelain

Mouth Outer Diameter 7.3 cm/ Belly Diameter 15.2 cm/ Bottom Diameter 8 cm/ Total Height Including the Lid 32.5 cm/ Belly Depth 23.2 cm/ Weight 2,300 g

带盖白釉瓶，用于盛装细药。

广东中医药博物馆藏

The jar with a lid is made of white glazed porcelain. It was utilized for containing fine medicine.

Preserved in Guangdong Chinese Medicine Museum

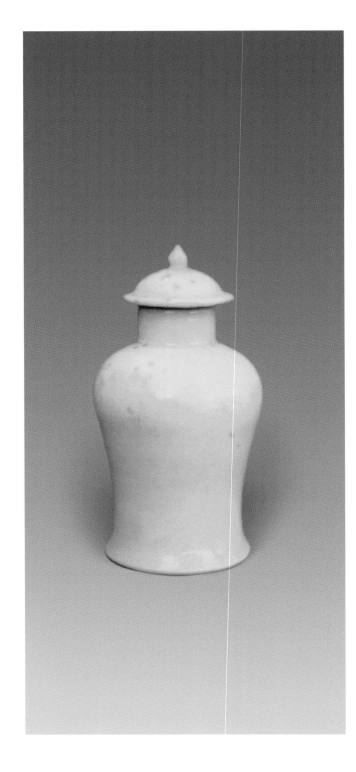

影青白瓷盖瓶

明

瓷质

口外径 4.19 厘米，最大腹径 8.74 厘米，底径 7.9 厘米，通高 16.97 厘米，腹深 12.8 厘米，重 410 克

Misty Blue White Porcelain Jar with Lid

Ming Dynasty

Porcelain

Mouth Outer Diameter 4.19 cm/ Maximum Belly Diameter 8.74 cm/ Bottom Diameter 7.9 cm/ Height 16.97 cm/ Belly Depth 12.8 cm/ Weight 410 g

直口，高领，圆肩，腹部上鼓，中部微束，平底，底边外侈，带盖，盖顶塔尖纽。用于盛装细药。

广东中医药博物馆藏

The porcelain medicine jar has a vertical mouth, a long neck, a round shoulder, a bulged and slightly tapered belly, and a flat bottom with a flared rim. The top of its lid is a pagoda-shaped knob. The jar was utilized for containing fine medicine.

Preserved in Guangdong Chinese Medicine Museum

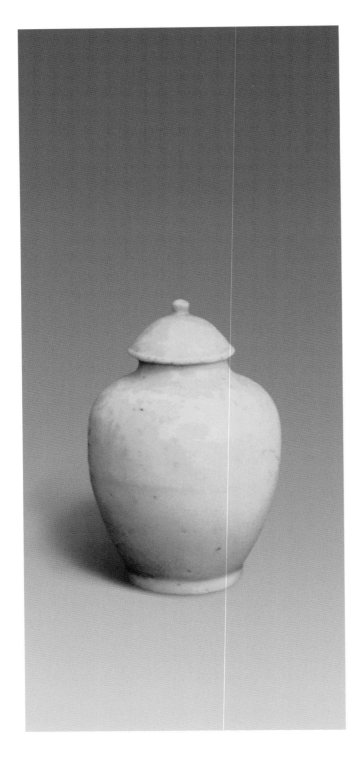

甜白盖瓶

明

瓷质

口外径 4.5 厘米，最大腹径 9.55 厘米，底径
6.1 厘米，通高 15 厘米，腹深 10.4 厘米，
重 395 克

Lovely White Porcelain Jar with Lid

Ming Dynasty

Porcelain

Mouth Outer Diameter 4.5 cm/ Maximum Belly
Diameter 9.55 cm/ Bottom Diameter 6.1 cm/ Height
15 cm/ Belly Depth 10.4 cm/ Weight 395 g

直口，腹上鼓下敛，平底，圈足，盖顶宝珠纽。
用于盛装细药。

广东中医药博物馆藏

The porcelain jar has a vertical mouth, a bulged
and tapered belly, a flat bottom, and a ring foot.
Its lid has a pearl-shaped knob. The jar was
utilized for containing fine medicine.
Preserved in Guangdong Chinese Medicine Museum

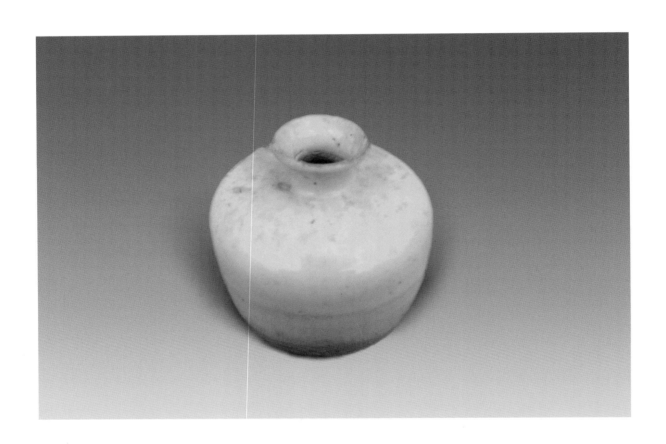

影青小口药瓶

明

瓷质

口外径 6.01 厘米， 腹径 14.13 厘米， 底径 12.05 厘米，通高 14.1 厘米，腹深 13.1 厘米，重 850 克

Misty Blue Medicine Bottle with Small Mouth

Ming Dynasty

Porcelain

Mouth Outer Diameter 6.01 cm/ Belly Diameter 14.13 cm/ Bottom Diameter 12.05 cm/ Height 14.1 cm/ Belly Depth 13.1 cm/ Weight 850 g

敞口，束颈，腹部上鼓下敛，平底。用于盛
装细药。

广东中医药博物馆藏

The porcelain medicine jar has a flared mouth, a
contracted neck, and a bulged and tapered belly.
It was utilized for containing fine medicine.
Preserved in Guangdong Chinese Medicine Museum

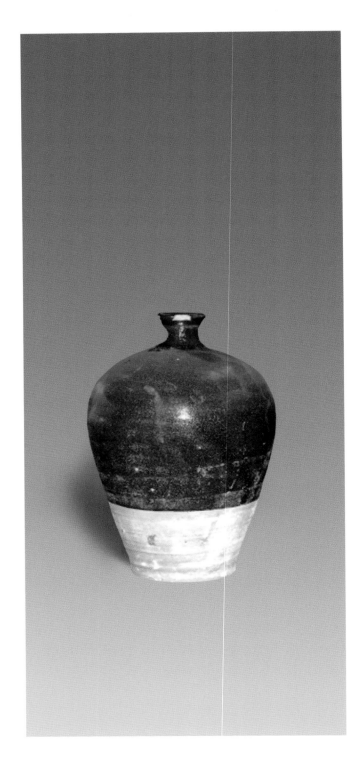

黑瓷瓶

明

瓷质

口径 4 厘米，底径 8.5 厘米，通高 22 厘米，

重 950 克

Black Porcelain Bottle

Ming Dynasty

Porcelain

Mouth Diameter 4 cm/ Bottom Diameter 8.5 cm/

Height 22 cm/ Weight 950 g

直口，高颈，圆肩，圆腹，圈足。下三分之
一无釉，白胎外露。为盛贮器。陕西历史博
物馆调拨。

陕西医史博物馆收藏

This bottle has a vertical mouth, a long neck, a round shoulder, a round belly and a ring foot. The lower one-third part is not coated with glaze, only showing the white body. The bottle was used for containing or storing things. It was allocated from Shaanxi History Museum.

Preserved in Shaanxi Museum of Medical History

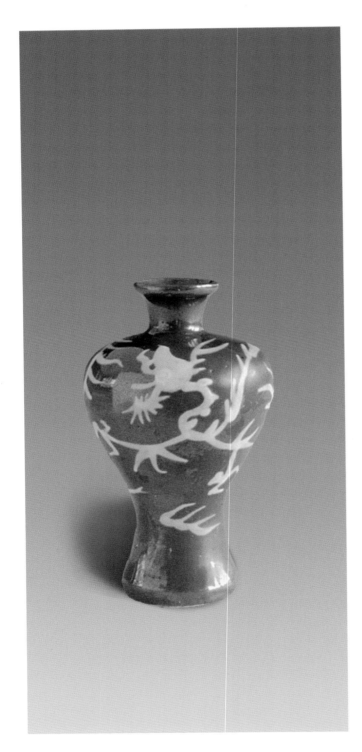

酱釉白龙纹梅瓶

明

瓷质

口径 3 厘米，底径 4 厘米，高 12 厘米

Brown Glazed Plum Vase with White Dragon Patterns

Ming Dynasty

Porcelain

Mouth Diameter 3 cm/ Bottom Diameter 4 cm/

Height 12 cm

浅盘口，短颈，丰肩，肩往下渐收至脚而外侈，
卧圈足。通体施酱釉，莹润光亮。身绘白釉
云龙纹，底施白釉。

蓝子杏藏

This vase has a shallow mouth, a short neck, a
plump shoulder, a contracted belly and a flared
ring foot. The body is covered with dark reddish
brown glaze, which is mellow and glossy. The
vase is decorated with among clouds dragon
patterns in white glaze. The bottom is also
covered with white glaze.
Collected by Lan Zixing

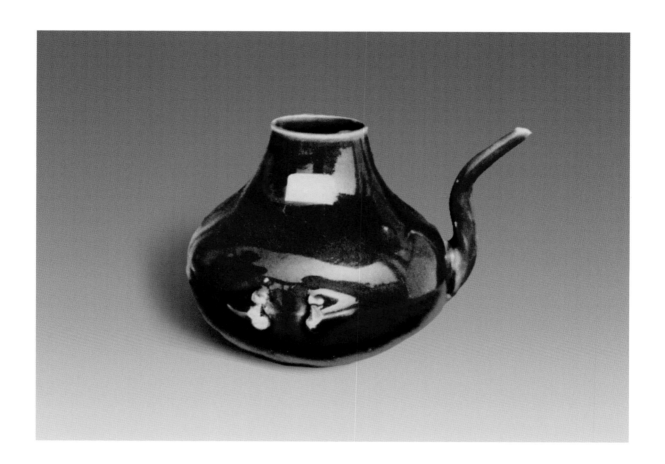

细嘴瓷壶

明

瓷质

腹径 13.6 厘米，高 11.9 厘米

Porcelain Pot with Small Mouth

Ming Dynasty

Porcelain

Belly Diameter 13.6 cm/ Height 11.9 cm

为药液淋洗眼疾之器具。江苏江阴夏颧墓
出土。

江阴博物馆藏

The porcelain pot was utilized for pouring
medicinal liquid into the eye to treat eye
diseases. It was unearthed from Xia Quan's
tomb in Jiangyin City, Jiangsu Province.

Preserved in Jiangyin Museum

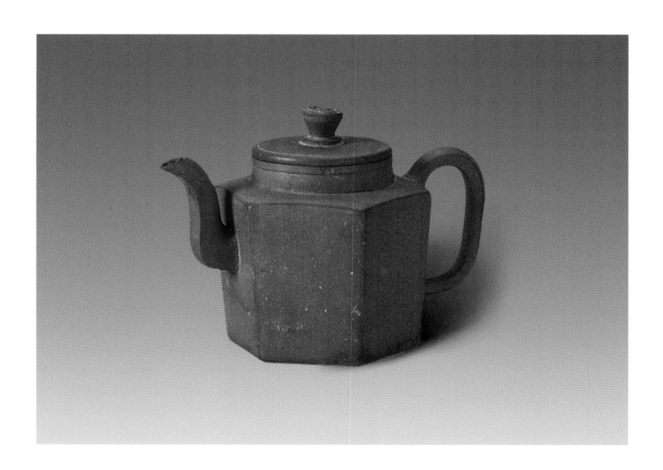

"大彬"款六方紫砂壶

明

紫砂质

通高 11 厘米

Dark Red Enameled Hexagonal Pottery Teapot Inscribed with "Da Bin"

Ming Dynasty

Dark Red Enameled Pottery

Height 11 cm

壶圆形盖，子口与壶口套合，盖顶圆纽，纽上印对合半弧纹。壶身六方形，直口，斜折肩，六棱形曲流，五角形弯执。底内凹，柴油砂泥质细润，色呈赭红，上有银砂闪点。底部正中刻"大彬"直行楷书款。1968年江苏江都县丁沟乡洪飞村郑王庄明墓出土。

扬州博物馆藏

The teapot has a round lid whose mouth matches the mouth of the teapot. On the top of the teapot there is a round knob decorated with merging arc patterns. The teapot has a hexagonal body, a vertical mouth, an inclined square shoulder, six-sided spout, a pentagonal bending handle, and a concave bottom. The clay belongs to fine diesel sand-mud and the color is reddish with silver flash spots. The center of the bottom is inscribed with two regular-script Chinese characters reading "Da Bin". The teapot was excavated from a Ming Dynasty tomb in Jiangdu County, Jiangsu Province, in 1968.
Preserved in Yangzhou Museum

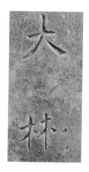
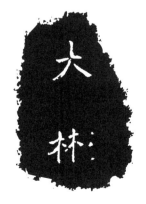

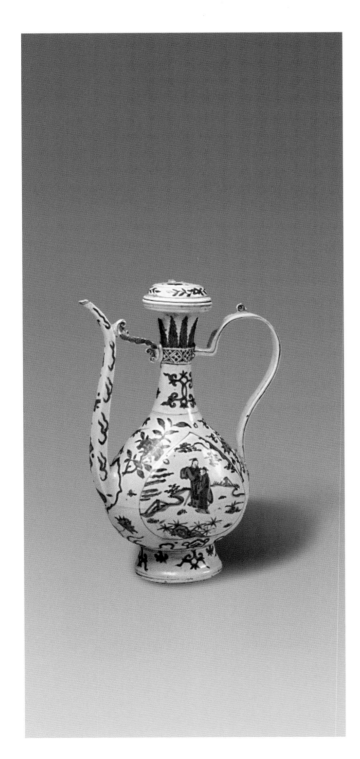

青花人物纹执壶

明

瓷质

口径 6.5 厘米，底径 8.4 厘米，通高 27.5 厘米

Blue-and-white Porcelain Pot Patterned with Figures

Ming Dynasty

Porcelain

Mouth Diameter 6.5 cm/ Bottom Diameter 8.4 cm/

Height 27.5 cm

子母口，细颈且长，扁圆腹，高圈足，柄和流弯曲且细长，盖面隆起有纽。胎细色白，釉白泛青色。遍体绘青花纹饰，腹部桃形开光内绘"野游图"和"松下听涛图"，线条流畅，人物神态自然。足内署青花楷书"福寿康宁"款。该壶属明嘉靖时期景德镇烧造。1967年山东招远市西吕家村出土。

招远市文物管理所藏

This pot has a snap-lid, a thin and long neck, an oblate belly, and a high ring foot. The handle and the spout are curved and elongated. There is a knob on the raised lid. The pot is covered with fine and white glaze suffused with blue. The surface is painted with blue-and-white patterns. The peach-shaped paneled part on the belly is painted with two pictures entitled "Excursion" and "Listening to Waves Under the Pine Tree", with smooth lines and natural expressions of the characters. On the foot are inscribed in blue-and-white regular script four Chinese characters reading "Fu Shou Kang Ning" (good fortune, long life, good health, and peacefulness). The pot was made in Jingdezhen kiln during Jiajing Period of the Ming Dynasty. It was excavated at western Lüjia Village in Zhaoyuan City, Shandong Province, in 1967.

Preserved in Zhaoyuan Municipal Administration Office of Cultural Relics

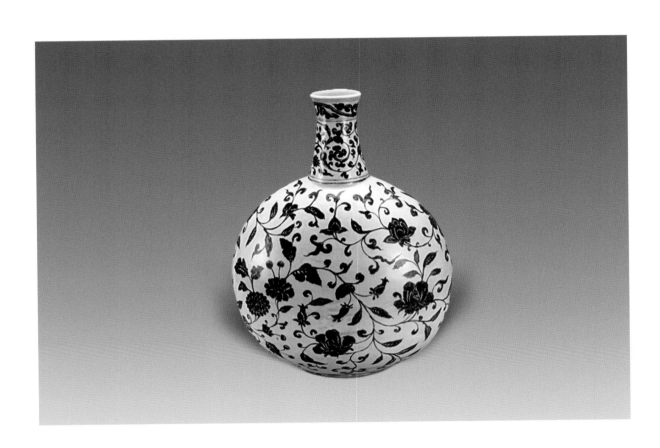

永乐青花缠枝莲纹扁壶

明

瓷质

口径 8.2 厘米，高 44 厘米

Blue-and-white Porcelain Oblate Pot Patterned with Intertwining Lotuses of Yongle Period

Ming Dynasty

Porcelain

Mouth Diameter 8.2 cm/ Height 44 cm

小口微侈，细颈，溜肩，扁鼓腹，圈足。胎质细腻纯净，白釉微泛青色。通体绘疏朗的青花纹饰。颈部两道纹饰分绘小缠枝莲花图案，腹部满绘勾莲的缠枝莲花，青花用料为苏泥勃青，色泽清晰明快，绚丽鲜艳，局部有结晶斑点，器型硕大，图案精美。为酒器。传世品。

扬州博物馆藏

This pot has a small and flared mouth, a thin neck, a narrow and inclined shoulder, an oblate and bulged belly, and a ring foot. The pottery body is fine and clear, the glaze is white suffused with blue. The surface is painted with sparse blue-and-white patterns. There are two patterns of small intertwining lotuses on the neck and connected intertwining lotuses on the belly. Smaltum paint was used to make the blue-and-white patterns which look distinct and bright. This pot is big and delicate with crystal spots. It was a drinking vessel which was a handed-down heirloom.

Preserved in Yangzhou Museum

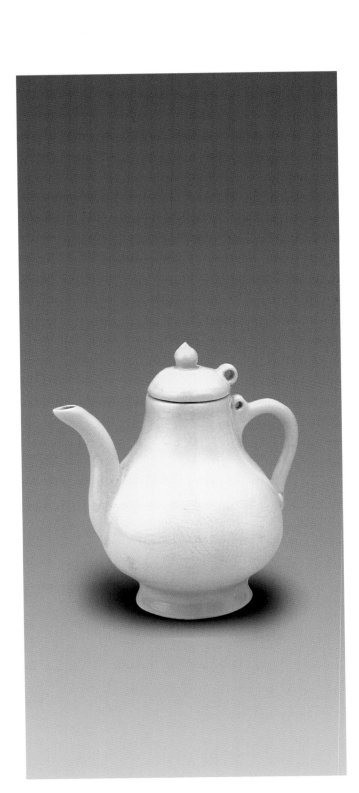

永乐甜白釉暗花凤纹梨式壶

明

瓷质

口径 4 厘米，底径 5.5 厘米，通高 12.5 厘米

White-glazed Pear-shaped Pot with Phoenix and Flower Patterns of Yongle Period

Ming Dynasty

Porcelain

Mouth Diameter 4 cm/ Bottom Diameter 5.5 cm/

Height 12.5 cm

壶形似鸭梨，流微曲，宝珠形盖纽，盖沿及柄上方各有一小系，圈足较高，外撇。通刻精细流畅的阴线暗花。盖面为覆莲纹，肩部刻4朵流云，腹部为一对回首展翅的凤凰，飘逸的凤尾配合巧妙地布置于凤体周转的数朵如意云纹；圈足的外侧饰有一圈云雷纹。该壶的胎质细腻、胎色洁白，满施甜白釉，釉较厚温润似玉。隐现极细的桔皮纹，足根露胎。为永乐瓷中的传世品精品。

扬州博物馆藏

The pot is shaped like a pear with a slightly tapered spout and a pearl-shaped knob. There is a small ring respectively on the lug and the edge of the lid. The high ring foot has a flared rim. The body is decorated with delicate veiled patterns. The lid is covered with lotus-petal designs. There are four clouds on the shoulder. The belly is painted with patterns of a pair of phoenixes looking back and spreading their wings surrounded by Ruyi-sceptre clouds. The outside of the ring foot is decorated with cloud and thunder patterns. Its sweet white glaze is as mellow as jade, faintly showing the fine orange-skin patterns. No glaze covers the bottom of the jar. This jar is a treasure that was handed down from Yongle Period of the Ming Dynasty for generations. Preserved in Yangzhou Museum

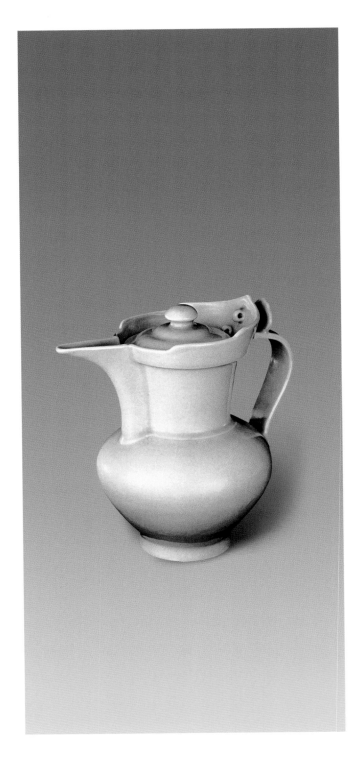

白釉僧帽壶

明

瓷质

流长 16.7 厘米，足径 7.5 厘米，高 19.7 厘米

壶上部略如僧帽，故称"僧帽壶"，流与颈
部流槽相通，柄上、下两端均呈如意形，绘
如意云头纹。腹上丰下窄。盖有纽。

故宫博物院藏

White-glazed Monk's Hat Pot

Ming Dynasty

Porcelain

Spout Length 16.7 cm/ Bottom Length 7.5 cm/
Height 19.7 cm

The upper part of the pot is shaped like a
monk's hat. The spout is connected with the
groove of the neck. Each end of the handle
is patterned with "Ruyi" clouds. The jar has a
bulged belly which tapers downwards and a
knob on the lid.

Preserved in The Palace Museum

赤地金彩童戏纹瓷碗

明

瓷质

口径 16.5 厘米

敞口，圜底，圈足。通体施红釉，碗壁内外用绿、金等色彩绘制童戏图案，其中的童子骑竹马游戏图情景生动，颇具生活韵味。

日本石川县立美术馆藏

Porcelain Bowl with Golden-colored Patterns on Red Background

Ming Dynasty

Porcelain

Mouth Diameter 16.5 cm

The bowl has a flared mouth, a round bottom, and a ring foot. The body is covered with red glaze. The interior and exterior walls of the bowl have patterns of playing boys painted with green and gold enamel. The scene of children riding bamboo horses is vivid and interesting.

Preserved in Ishikawa Prefectural Museum of Art, Japan

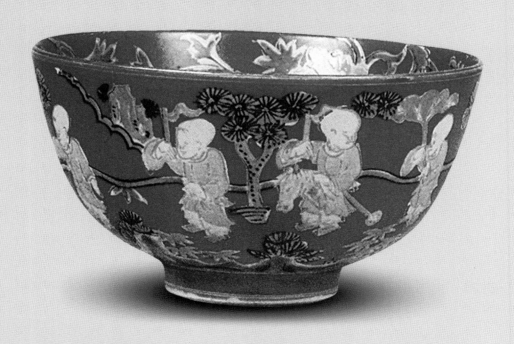

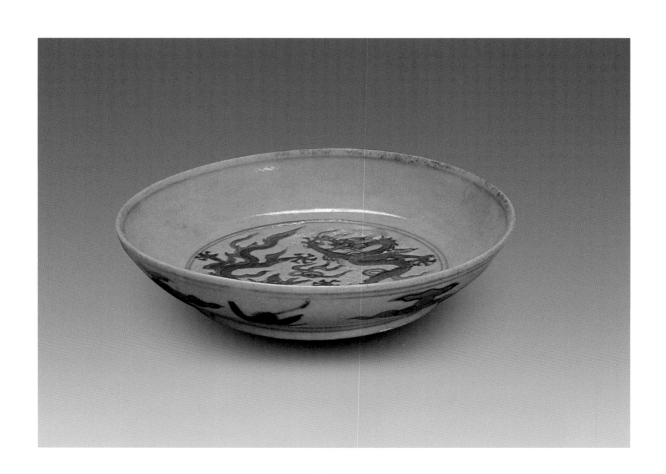

黄地五彩云鹤纹碗

明

瓷质

高 3.1 厘米

Multi-colored Porcelain Bowl with Cranes and Clouds on Yellow Background

Ming Dynasty

Porcelain

Height 3.1 cm

敞口，浅腹，圈足。盘内、外及底均施黄釉，
盘心绘双龙戏珠，一降龙用青料绘成，一升龙
用红彩绘成。盘外壁用青料绘四仙鹤，用红彩
绘四云纹，相间配置。盘底暗刻双圈双行"大
明万历年制"书款。胎体薄匀，制作规整，在
万历彩瓷中属上乘之作。

南京市博物馆藏

The bowl has a flared mouth, a shallow belly, and a ring foot. Its interior, exterior and bottom are covered with yellow glaze. Its center is painted with patterns of two dragons playing with a pearl. The descending and the ascending dragons are respectively painted blue and red. The exterior wall of the bowl is decorated alternately with four cranes and four clouds painted respectively with cobalt blue pigment and red pigment. The bottom of the bowl is inscribed with a six-character seal mark reading "Da Ming Wan Li Nian Zhi" (made during Wanli Period of the Ming Dynasty). The pottery body is thin and homogeneous and the styling is well-structured. The collection is one of the best among the colored porcelain works made during Wanli Period.

Preserved in Nanjing Municipal Museum

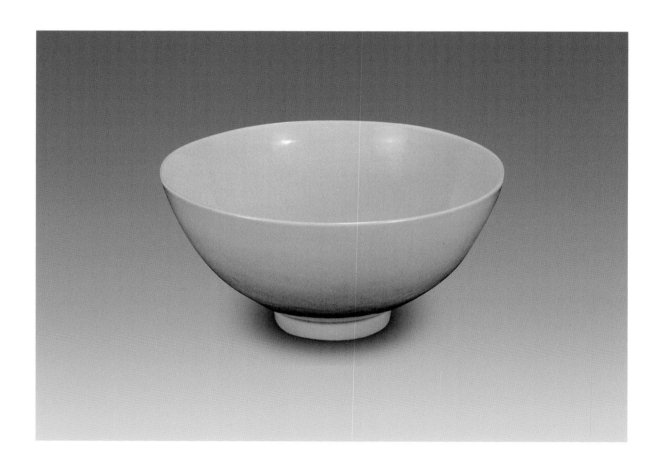

永乐白釉暗花大碗

明

瓷质

口径 21 厘米，底径 7.4 厘米，高 10.2 厘米

White-glazed Bowl with Flower Patterns of Yongle Period

Ming Dynasty

Porcelain

Mouth Diameter 21 cm/ Bottom Diameter 7.4 cm/ Height 10.2 cm

敞口，深腹斜壁，圈足。胎洁白细腻，内、外均施白釉，釉面光亮莹润。内壁口沿阴刻草叶纹一周，腹部阴刻莲瓣纹。外壁口沿阴刻回纹一周，腹部刻缠枝花卉。

河北博物院藏

This plate has a flared mouth, a deep and sloping belly, a ring foot, and white and fine pottery body. The interior wall is carved with a cirle of grass and leaf patterns on its mouth rim and lotus petal patterns on the belly. The exterior wall is carved with a circle of fret patterns on its mouth rim and intertwining branches on the belly.

Preserved in Hebei Museum

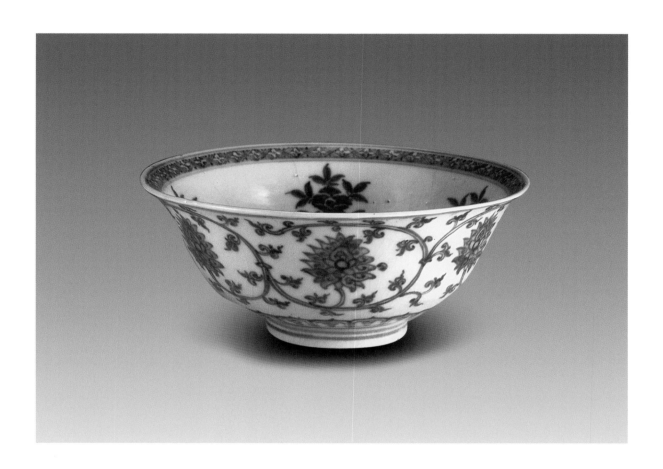

成化青花缠枝莲纹碗

明

瓷质

口径 19.8 厘米，底径 7.2 厘米，高 8.5 厘米

Blue-and-white Bowl Patterned with Intertwining Lotus Branches of Chenghua Period

Ming Dynasty

Porcelain

Mouth Diameter 19.8 cm/ Bottom Diameter 7.2 cm/ Height 8.5 cm

碗口沿外撇，壁微弧，圈足内敛，内、外壁均绘青花纹饰。内底心饰如意结带宝杵纹，内壁绘一周5朵折枝山茶花，内沿绘一周锦纹带，外口沿饰双弦纹，腹部以大朵缠枝莲花为主体装饰，下绘一周莲瓣纹，内壁花卉为没骨画法，外壁花卉采用双勾平涂技法绘制，构图独具匠心。胎质轻薄细白而紧密；釉面肥厚滋润，光洁无瑕，釉色呈淡淡的湖水青；造型精巧俊秀，青花色调恬静雅致。1978年扬州市农业科学研究所明墓出土。

扬州博物馆藏

The mouth of the bowl is flared. The body is a little crooked and the ring foot is tapered. The interior and exterior walls are painted with blue-and-white decorations. The inner bottom is painted with Ruyi-sceptre knotted bands with pestle designs. The interior wall is decorated with five plucked camellia branches painted with the technique "outlined painting". The inside and outside of the rim are painted with brocade and bow string designs. The principal motif is big intertwining lotuses, under which are a circle of lotus petal designs. The traditional technique "outline sketch and coloring" was utilized on the exterior wall. The composition is unique. The pottery body is light and thin, white and fine. The lake-colored green glaze is bright and clean, tranquil and graceful without flaws. It is a work with fine craftsmanship. The artifact was excavated from a tomb of the Ming Dynasty by Yangzhou Institute of Agricultural Sciences in 1978.

Preserved in Yangzhou Museum

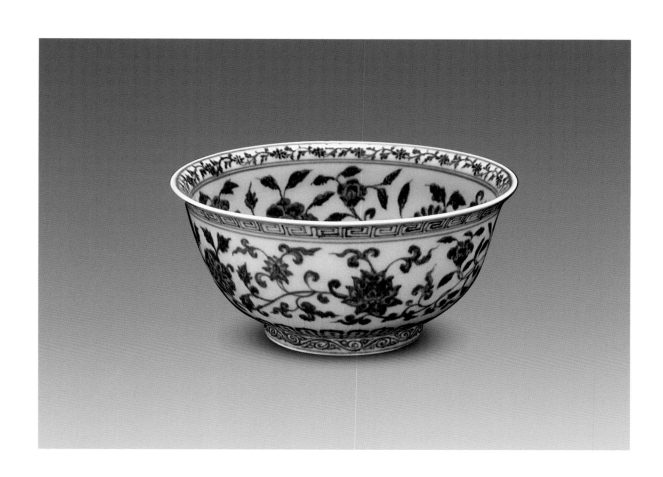

青花缠枝莲纹碗

明

瓷质

口径 19.4 厘米，底径 9.1 厘米，高 19.4 厘米

Blue-and-white Bowl Patterned with Winding Lotus Branches

Ming Dynasty

Porcelain

Mouth Diameter 19.4 cm/ Bottom Diameter 9.1 cm/ Height 19.4 cm

敞口，深腹，壁微鼓，圈足。胎洁白致密，
釉色白中闪青，釉面光亮润泽。外壁口沿饰
回纹，腹部饰缠枝莲，近足部绘莲瓣纹和海
水纹。内壁口沿饰缠枝灵芝，腹部及内底绘
缠枝莲花。

河北博物院藏

The porcelain bowl has a flared mouth, a deep
and bulged belly, and a ring foot. The pottery
body is white and fine. The glaze is lustrous
and white with a glaucous tinge. The rim of
the exterior wall is decorated with fret patterns
while the belly is painted with intertwining lotus
branches. The foot is painted with patterns of
lotus-petal and waves. The rim of the interior
wall is decorated with winding gonaderma
branches. The intertwining lotus branches were
drawn on the belly and inner bottom.

Preserved in Hebei Museum

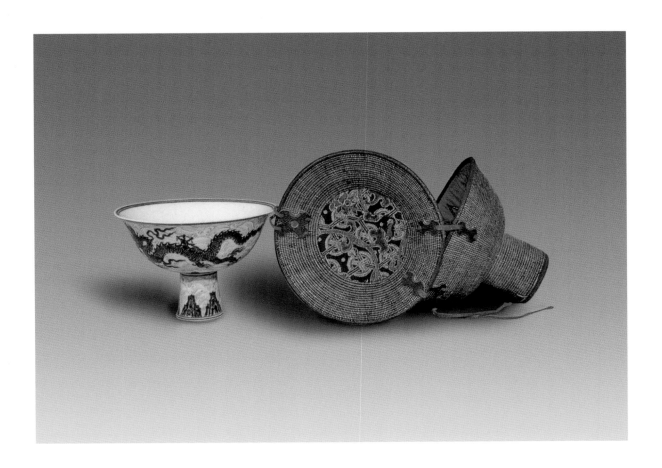

青花双龙高足碗

明

瓷质

口径 15.7 厘米，底径 4.69 厘米，高 10.7 厘米

Blue-and-white High-footed Bowl with Two Dragons

Ming Dynasty

Porcelain

Mouth Diameter 15.7 cm/ Bottom Diameter 4.69 cm/ Height 10.7 cm

敞口，圜底，高圈足，带碗套。通体白釉，
器壁绘青花龙纹。为明宣德年间制品。

西藏博物馆藏

The bowl has a flared mouth, a round bottom,
a high ring foot, and a case. The whole body is
covered with white glaze. The wall is painted
with blue-and-white dragon designs. The bowl
was made during Xuande Period of the Ming
Dynasty.

Preserved in Tibet Museum

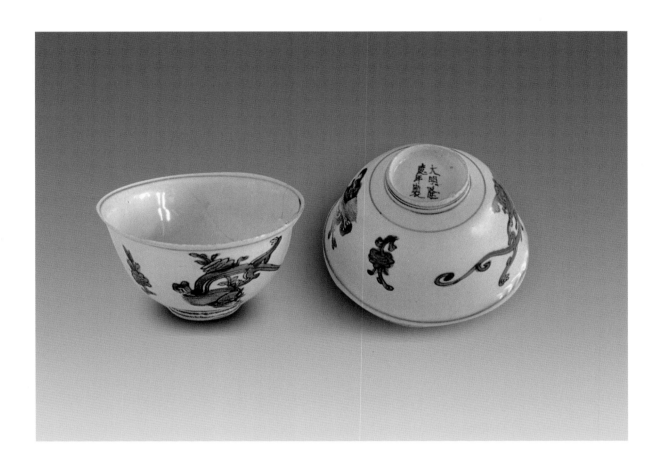

青花龙纹碗

明

瓷质

口径 9.5 厘米

Blue-and-white Bowl with Dragon Designs

Ming Dynasty

Porcelain

Mouth Diameter 9.5 cm

口撇略折，深腹，圈足。外壁绘花卉，夔龙纹，青花鲜艳，微微闪紫。底书写"大明隆庆年制"六字楷书款。

潘锡九藏

The porcelain bowl has a flared and folded rim, a deep belly, and a ring foot. The exterior wall of the bowl is decorated with flower and Kui-dragon patterns. The color of blue-and-white is brilliant with smacks of purple. The bottom of the bowl is inscribed with six characters reading "Da Ming Long Qing Nian Zhi" (made during Longqing Period of the Ming Dynasty) in regular script.

Collected by Pan Xijiu

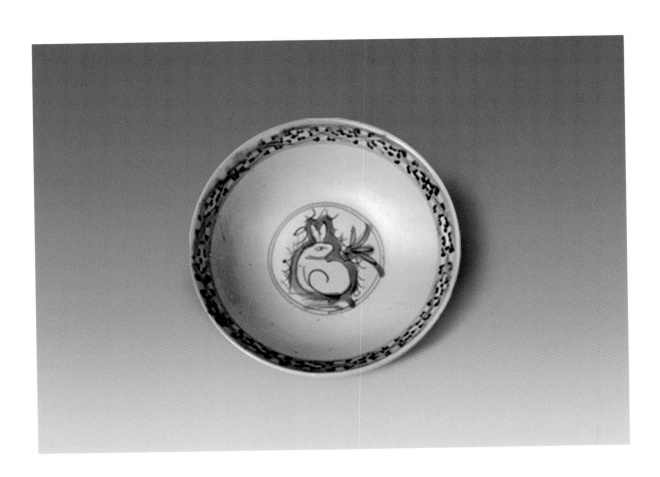

青花兔纹碗

明

瓷质

口径 12.8 厘米，底径 5.6 厘米，高 4 厘米

Blue-and-white Bowl with Rabbit Patterns

Ming Dynasty

Porcelain

Mouth Diameter 12.8 cm/ Bottom Diameter 5.6 cm/ Height 4 cm

敞口，深腹，圈足。通体白釉青花，内壁口缘绘斜榄状纹及点纹，碗中央绘花卉，其间有一只竖耳昂首的卧兔，用笔简练，画意传神，是民间艺人的佳作。青花色鲜艳，闪淡的紫色，白釉莹润闪青，是万历年间作品。

梁万程藏

The bowl has a flared mouth, a deep belly, and a ring foot. The whole body is covered with white-glazed blue-and-white. The rim of the interior wall is painted with oblique olive and dot patterns. The center of the bowl is decorated with floral designs, in which there is a crouching rabbit with erecting ears and a raising head. The strokes are simple and expressive. The bowl was one of the masterpieces made by folk artists. The color of blue-and-white is bright with smacks of purple. The glaze is white with a glaucous tinge. The artifact was produced during Wanli Period of the Ming Dynasty. Collected by Liang Wancheng

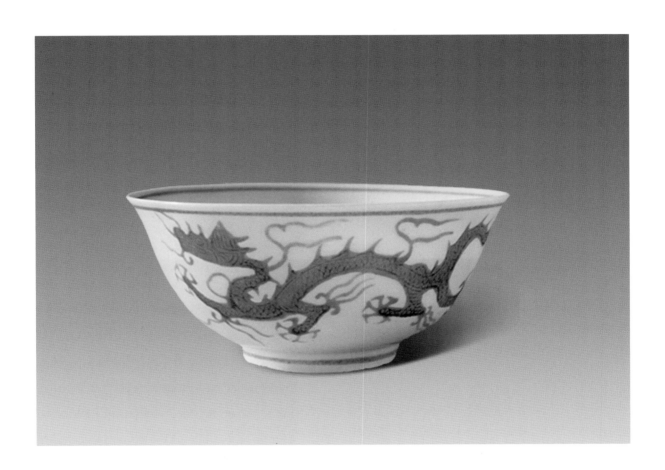

白釉绿龙纹碗

明

瓷质

口径 18.6 厘米

White-glazed Bowl with Green Dragon Patterns

Ming Dynasty

Porcelain

Mouth Diameter 18.6 cm

敞口，深腹，圈足。内壁口缘绘弦纹，外壁绘对称的绿釉龙纹，是先在素胎面上刻划出轮廓线，然后加绘绿釉在其上面。外口缘及足处各绘一周绿釉弦纹，底用青花书写"大明正德年制"六字楷书双圈款。碗壁绿釉莹润，是正德年间宫廷用品。

高丰藏

The porcelain bowl has a flared mouth, a deep belly, and a ring foot. The rim of the interior wall is painted with bow string patterns. The exterior wall is painted with patterns of two green-glazed dragons. The technique involved was drawing the outline on the biscuit first and then covering it with green glaze. The external rim and the foot are painted with green-glazed bow string patterns. The bottom of the bowl is inscribed with six characters reading "Da Ming Zheng De Nian Zhi" (made during Zhengde Period of the Ming Dynasty) in regular script surrounded by double circles. The bowl was an imperial utensil during Zhengde Period of the Ming Dynasty.

Collected by Gao Feng

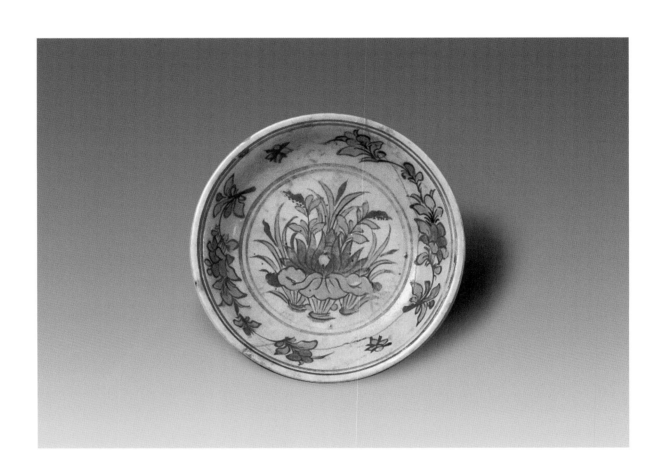

五彩莲花盘

明

瓷质

口径 15 厘米，底径 8 厘米，高 3.3 厘米

Multi-colored Plate with Lotus Patterns

Ming Dynasty

Porcelain

Mouth Diameter 15 cm/ Bottom Diameter 8 cm/ Height 3.3 cm

敞口，浅腹，平底，圈足，内、外施白釉。釉上用红、绿、黄彩绘画图案，盘心饰莲花与水草，内壁折枝桃花，外壁饰折枝牡丹。底足内红彩楷书"福"字款。此盘为釉上五彩瓷早期作品，是弘治年间景德镇民窑烧制。

兖州博物馆藏

The plate has a flared mouth, a shallow belly, a flat bottom, and a ring foot. The interior and exterior are covered with white glaze, on which there are red, green and yellow patterns. The center of the plate is decorated with patterns of lotus and aquatic plants; the interior and exterior walls are respectively patterned with plucked peach branches and plucked peony branches. There is an regular-script Chinese character reading "Fu" (blessing) written in red color on the bottom. This plate belonged to the works of early-stage overglaze five-colored porcelain. It was made by a folk kiln in Jingdezhen during Hongzhi Period of the Ming Dynasty.

Preserved in Yanzhou Museum

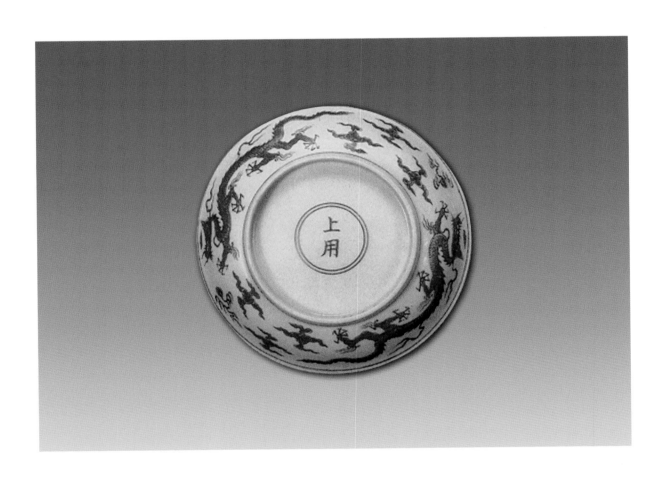

红彩龙纹盘

明

瓷质

口径 20 厘米，底径 13.5 厘米，高 4.5 厘米

Red-enamelled Plate with Dragon Patterns

Ming Dynasty

Porcelain

Mouth Diameter 20 cm/ Bottom Diameter 13.5 cm/ Height 4.5 cm

盘弧壁带矮圈足。内壁釉色洁白，光亮如镜。外壁在白底上用红彩绘出双龙戏珠图案。此盘为明弘治年间制品，胎体较薄，红彩深沉而不失艳丽，制作规整，是明代釉里红瓷器的精品。盘底正中，在红色双圈之内，有工整的楷书"上用"二字，明确地标示出此盘是皇帝御用食具。

故宫博物院藏

The plate has a cambered wall and a short ring foot. It is covered with white glaze which is like a shining mirror. The exterior wall is painted with patterns of two dragons playing with a pearl in red enamel against the white background. The plate, which was made in Hongzhi Period of the Ming Dynasty, has thin pottery body. Red enamel color is deep but bright. The plate is a masterpiece of underglaze red porcelain ware with well-structured styling. In the red circle of the bottom center, there are two characters reading "Shang Yong" in regular script, indicating that the plate was an imperial tableware.

Preserved in The Palace Museum

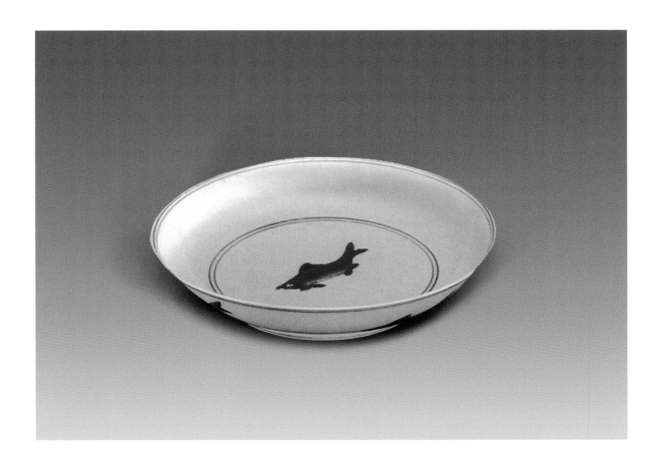

矾红鱼纹盘

明

瓷质

口径 17.7 厘米，高 3.8 厘米

Orangish Red Plate with Fish Patterns

Ming Dynasty

Porcelain

Mouth Diameter 17.7 cm/ Height 3.8 cm

敞口，浅腹，矮圈足。口沿内、外及内底和
足部各饰两周红彩弦纹，并在盘心双圈内用
矾红绘出一尾红鱼，外壁绘四条。胎釉洁白
纯正，红色艳丽生动，图案疏密有致，层次
分明，生活气息浓郁。明嘉靖年间制品。

首都博物馆藏

The plate has a flared mouth, a shallow belly,
and a short ring foot. The rim, interior bottom
and foot are respectively painted with two
circles of red bow string patterns. An orangish
red fish is painted within the double circles in
the center of the plate and four fishes on the
exterior wall. The pottery body and glaze are
pure white. The red color is bright and lively.
The patterns are arranged with proper density
and distinct gradation. The plate, which shows
strong vitality, was made during Jiajing Period
of the Ming Dynasty.
Preserved in The Capital Museum

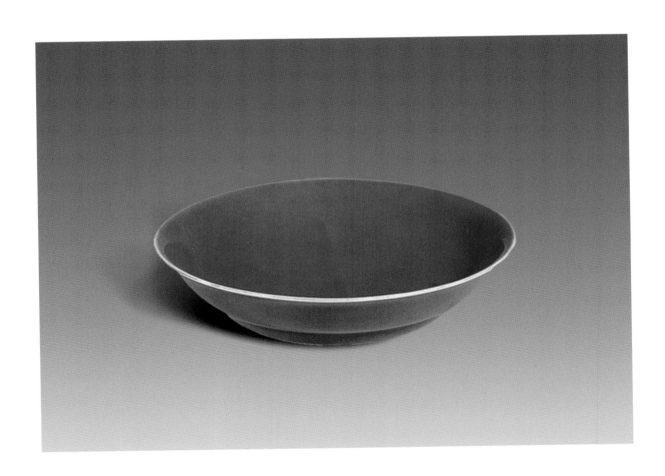

宣德红釉盘

明

瓷质

口径 21.4 厘米，底径 13.1 厘米，高 4.3 厘米

Red-glazed Plate of Xuande Period

Ming Dynasty

Porcelain

Mouth Diameter 21.4 cm/ Bottom Diameter 13.1 cm/ Height 4.3 cm

敞口，弧壁，大圈足。胎洁白细腻，内、外均施红釉，釉面肥厚润泽。口沿呈透明的白色釉，俗称"灯草口"。底书青花双圈"大明宣德年制"六字两行楷书款。

河北博物院藏

The plate has a flared mouth, a cambered wall, and a big ring foot. The pottery body is white and fine. The plate is covered with red lustrous glaze except for the rim which is coated with transparent white glaze. The bottom of the plate is inscribed with six characters reading "Da Ming Xuan De Nian Zhi" (made during Xuande Period of the Ming Dynasty) which are written in regular script and surrounded by double blue-and-white circles.

Preserved in Hebei Museum

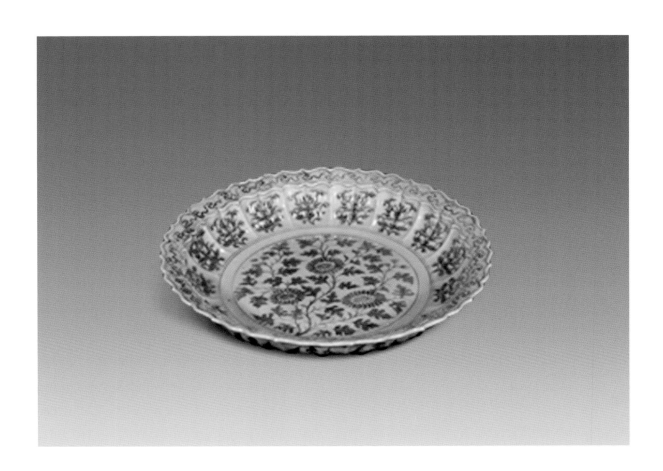

釉里红折枝菊纹菱花形盘

明

瓷质

口径 45.9 厘米，底径 27.7 厘米，高 8.6 厘米

Underglaze Plate Patterned with Red Plucked Chrysanthemum Branches

Ming Dynasty

Porcelain

Mouth Diameter 45.9 cm/ Bottom Diameter 27.7 cm/ Height 8.6 cm

菱花形口，花瓣形浅腹，矮圈足。胎洁白细腻，

釉色白中微闪青，盘底绘折枝菊花图案。

河北博物院藏

The plate has a Ryoka-shaped mouth, a petal-shaped shallow belly, and short ring foot. The pottery body is white and a fine. The glaze is white with a glaucous tinge. The bottom of the plate is painted with patterns of plucked chrysanthemum branches.

Preserved in Hebei Museum

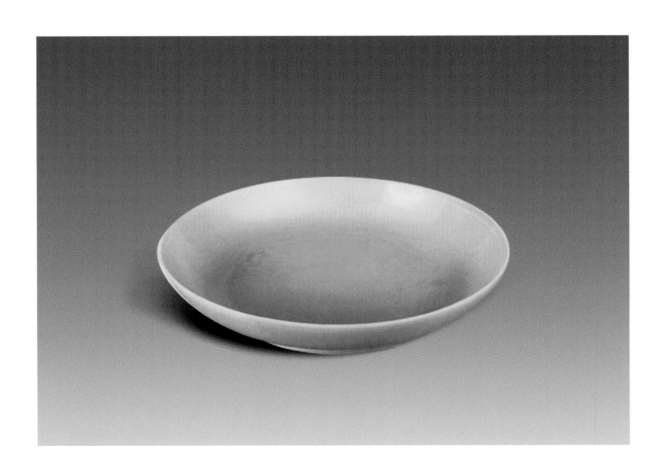

黄釉盘

明

瓷质

口径 21.2 厘米，底径 13.3 厘米，高 4.4 厘米

Yellow-glazed Plate

Ming Dynasty

Porcelain

Mouth Diameter 21.2 cm/ Bottom Diameter 13.3 cm/ Height 4.4 cm

圆唇，曲腹，器表施一层黄釉，底部有青花楷书"大明弘治年制"的题款。釉层肥厚，釉色黄嫩，是明弘治年间娇黄釉瓷器的典型作品。

北京大学赛克勒考古与艺术博物馆藏

The plate has a circular mouth and a cambered belly. Its surface is covered with thick and yellow glaze. The bottom of the plate is inscribed with six characters reading "Da Ming Hong Zhi Nian Zhi" (made during Hongzhi Period of the Ming Dynasty) in blue-and-white regular script. The plate is typical of masterpieces of bright yellow porcelain ware in Hongzhi Period of the Ming Dynasty.

Preserved in The Arthur M. Sackler Museum of Art and Archaeology at Peking University

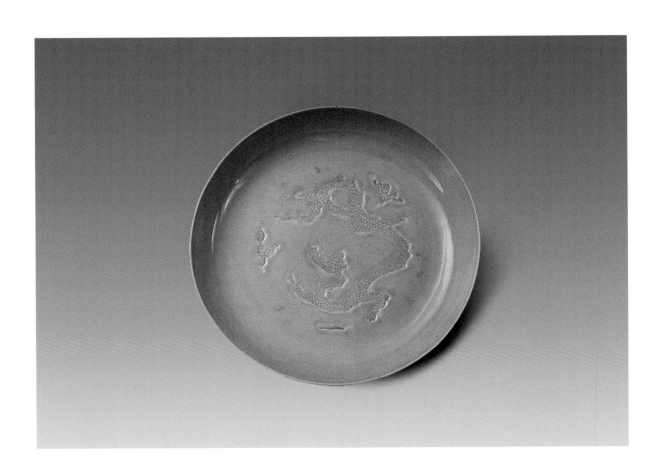

青白釉云龙纹盘

明

瓷质

口径 22.6 厘米，底径 14.5 厘米，高 4.5 厘米

Greenish White-glazed Plate with Dragon and Cloud Designs

Ming Dynasty

Porcelain

Mouth Diameter 22.6 cm/ Bottom Diameter 14.5 cm/ Height 4.5 cm

口微敛，浅腹，底近平，圈足。胎薄，质细，色洁白。内、外施釉肥润，白中闪青色。在内底胎上刻画一团龙，衬以云纹，外壁刻画双行龙及云朵。刻纹处露胎未施釉，因胎中铁粒氧化而呈现赭色。底有青花楷书"大明正德年制"款。饰纹设计新颖，制作精巧。

青岛市博物馆藏

The plate has a slightly contracted mouth, a shallow belly, a flat bottom, and a ring foot. The pottery body is pure white, thin and fine. The interior and exterior are coated with thick and lustrous white glaze with a glaucous tinge. There is a dragon surrounded by clouds carved in the interior bottom of the plate. The exterior wall is incised with two rows of dragons and clouds. The carved pattern is not covered with glaze, showing sienna because of the oxidization of iron. The bottom of the plate is inscribed with six characters reading "Da Ming Zheng De Nian Zhi" (made during Zhengde Period of the Ming Dynasty) in regular script. The plate shows unique designs and delicate workmanship.

Preserved in Qingdao Municipal Museum

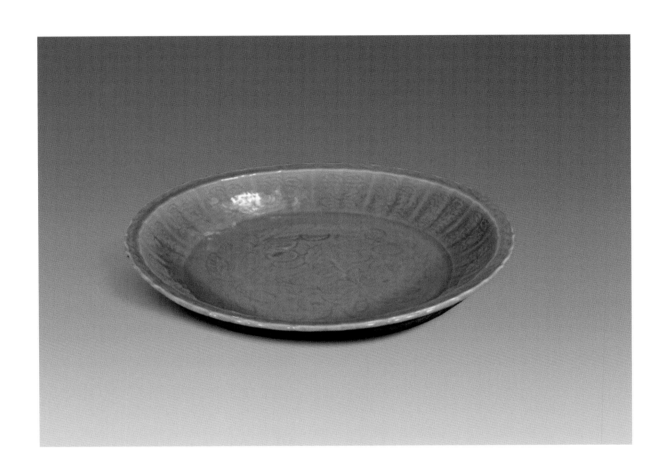

龙泉窑青釉折枝荔枝纹花口大盘

明

瓷质

口径 55.3 厘米，高 9.8 厘米

Big Celadon Plate with Flower-shaped Mouth and Litchi Patterns

Ming Dynasty

Porcelain

Mouth Diameter 55.3 cm/ Height 9.8 cm

菱花口，折沿，浅腹，矮圈足。胎体洁白细腻，厚重，内、外施满豆青釉，釉色浮光明显，玻化程度高。内壁刻画折枝莲，盘底刻折枝荔枝，器形硕大。

河北博物院藏

This big plate has a Ryoka-shaped mouth, a flared and flat rim, a shallow belly, and a short ring foot. The pottery body is white, fine and thick. The interior and exterior of the plate are covered with light bluish green glaze, shiny and highly vitrified. The interior wall is carved with a plucked lotus. The bottom of the big plate is incised with plucked litchi branches.

Preserved in Hebei Museum

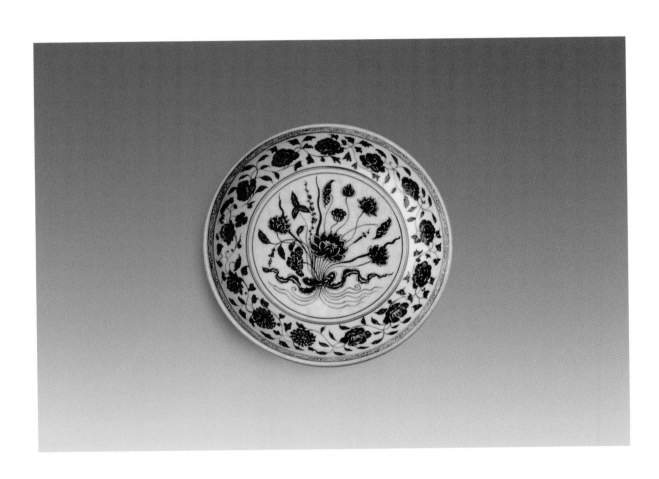

青花束莲盘

明

瓷质

口径 28.3 厘米，底径 20.5 厘米，高 5.4 厘米

Blue-and-white Plate with Lotus Bunches

Ming Dynasty

Porcelain

Mouth Diameter 28.3 cm/ Bottom Diameter 20.5 cm/ Height 5.4 cm

盘浅腹平底，有矮圈足。胎质细腻洁白，通
体施釉，底足露胎。盘底白胎上用进口钴料
绘出蓝色花卉图案，边饰则用国产钴料绘制
花卉图案，然后罩上一层亮度极高的透明釉，
釉层纯净匀称。这种色泽搭配，使主题纹样
更加突出。明宣德年间制品。

北京大学赛克勒考古与艺术博物馆藏

The plate has a shallow belly, a flat bottom,
and a short ring foot. The pottery body is fine
and white. The plate is covered with glaze
except for the bottom and the foot. Blue flower
patterns are painted on the center of the plate
with imported cobalt and flower designs are
drawn around the rim with domestic cobalt, on
which there is a layer of pure, even and extreme
high-gloss glaze. This kind of color collocation
highlights the principal motif. The plate was
made during Xuande Period of the Ming
Dynasty.

Preserved in The Arthur M. Sackler Museum of
Art and Archaeology at Peking University

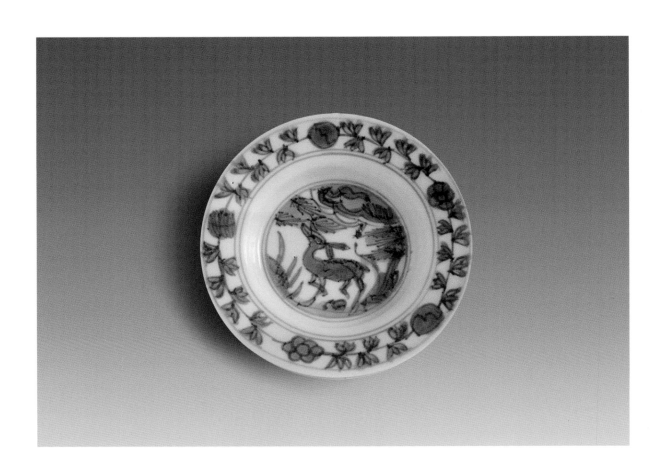

青花鹿纹碟

明

瓷质

口径 9.5 厘米，底径 4.8 厘米，高 2 厘米

Blue-and-white Dish with Deer Patterns

Ming Dynasty

Porcelain

Mouth Diameter 9.5 cm/ Bottom Diameter 4.8 cm/ Height 2 cm

折缘浅腹，圈足。碟内口缘绘缠枝花卉，中央绘松鹿纹，鹿正提一前蹄一后腿，伸颈抬首张望前方，似略有所闻状，底用青花书写"大明万历年制"楷书双圈款，青花呈色鲜艳，有闪淡紫色倾向，应是万历中后期作品。

钟汝更藏

The dish has a folded rim, a shallow belly, and a ring foot. The inner rim is painted with intertwining branches. The center of the dish is decorated with a deer that is looking into the distance with its foreleg, hind leg and head raised, appearing to be sniffing. The bottom of the dish is inscribed with six characters reading "Da Ming Wan Li Nian Zhi" (made during Wanli Period of the Ming Dynasty) which are written in regular script and surrounded by double blue-and-white circles. The blue-and-white is bright with a tinge of light purple. The dish should be a production in mid and late Wanli Period.

Collected by Zhong Rugeng

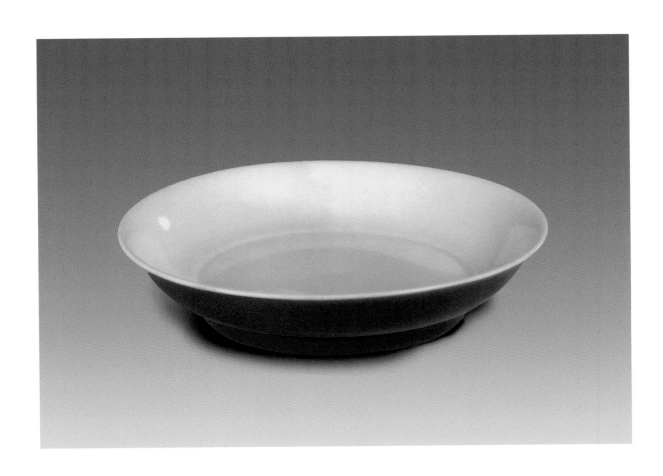

宣德蓝釉盘

明

瓷质

口径 20.3 厘米，底径 12.9 厘米，高 4.6 厘米

Blue-glazed Plate of Xuande Period

Ming Dynasty

Porcelain

Mouth Diameter 20.3 cm/ Bottom Diameter 12.9 cm/ Height 4.6 cm

敞口，浅腹弧壁，大圈足。胎洁白细腻，外壁施蓝釉，内壁及底施白釉。底书青花双圈"大明宣德年制"六字双行楷书款。釉色莹润光亮，造型端庄稳重。

河北博物院藏

The plate has a flared mouth, a shallow belly, and a big ring foot. The pottery body is white and fine. Its exterior wall is covered with blue glaze while the interior wall and the bottom are coated with glaze. The bottom of the plate is inscribed with six characters reading "Da Ming Xuan De Nian Zhi" (made during Xuande Period of the Ming Dynasty) which are written in regular script and surrounded by double blue-and-white circles. The glaze is lustrous and bright. The style of the plate is elegant.

Preserved in Hebei Museum

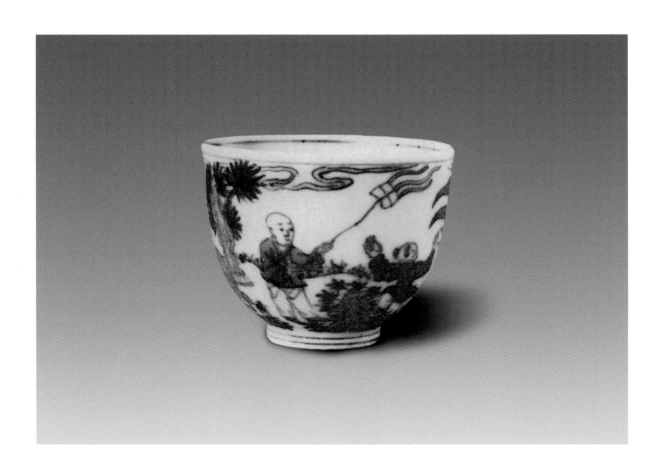

斗彩风筝纹瓷杯

明

瓷质

口径 6 厘米，高 4.8 厘米

Clashing-colored Cup with Kite Patterns

Ming Dynasty

Porcelain

Mouth Diameter 6 cm/ Height 4.8 cm

直口，深腹，圈足。杯外壁绘有童子于野外
放风筝的图案，筝线牵于一童子手内，风筝
已飘往空中，旁有一童子边遥望着风筝，边
手舞足蹈。画面活泼生动。

故宫博物院藏

The cup has a vertical mouth, a deep belly, and
a ring foot. The exterior wall is decorated with
a scene of children flying kites. The kite thread
is held in a boy's hand and the kite is flying
high in the sky. Another boy is looking at the
kite, waving his hand and dancing. The scene is
lively and vivid.

Preserved in The Palace Museum

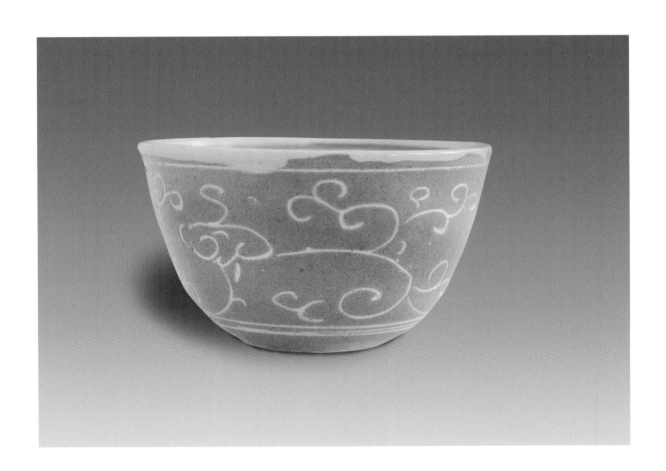

酱色釉刻花杯

明

瓷质

口径 8.5 厘米

Dark Reddish Brown-glazed Cup with Carved Flower Patterns

Ming Dynasty

Porcelain

Mouth Diameter 8.5 cm

敞口，深腹，卧足。外施酱色釉，刻画卷草纹，

刀法简练流畅。内施白釉，莹润，厚处闪青。

底用青花书写"大明年造"四字款。

邓其根藏

The cup has a flared mouth, a deep belly, and a concave foot. Its surface is covered with dark reddish brown glaze and decorated with scroll design. The way of cutting is simple and smooth. The interior of the cup is covered with white glaze which is lustrous with a glaucous tinge. The bottom of the cup is inscribed with four characters reading "Da Ming Nian Zao" (made in the Ming Dynasty) in blue-and-white.

Collected by Deng Qigen

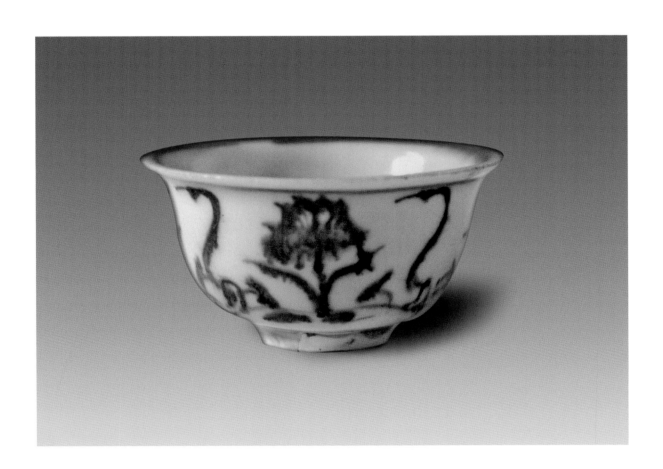

青花荷花纹杯

明

瓷质

口径 7.3 厘米，底径 2.8 厘米，高 3.9 厘米

Blue-and-white Cup with Lotus Patterns

Ming Dynasty

Porcelain

Mouth Diameter 7.3 cm/ Bottom Diameter 2.8 cm/ Height 3.9 cm

折沿，深腹，圈足。外壁绘荷花水藻纹，内壁中央绘寿山福海图，底用青花写"大明年造"四字。

招煊藏

The cup has a folded rim, a deep belly, and a ring foot. The exterior wall is decorated with lotus and algae patterns. The inner center is decorated with the picture of mountains and seas. The bottom of the cup is inscribed with four characters reading "Da Ming Nian Zao" (made in the Ming Dynasty) in blue-and-white. Collected by Zhao Xuan

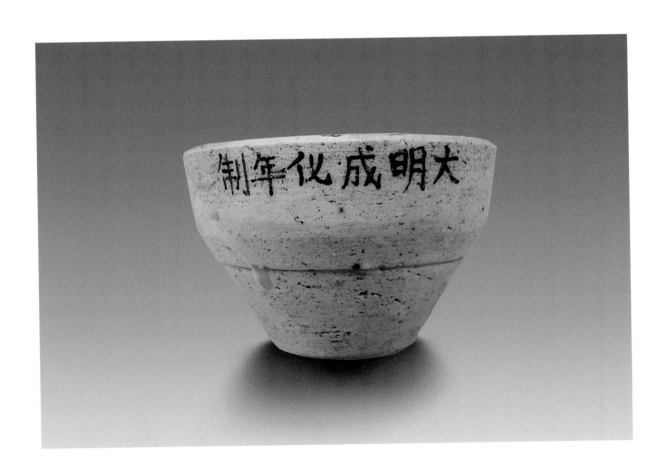

煎参汤杯

明

瓷质

口径 7 厘米，高 4.9 厘米

Ginseng Soup Slow-boiling Cup

Ming Dynasty

Porcelain

Mouth Diameter 7 cm/ Height 4.9 cm

敞口，圆唇，折腹，下腹斜收，平底。瓷质粗糙。
口沿下部墨书"大明成化年制"。

张雅宗藏

The cup, with crude texture, has a flared mouth, a round rim and a folded belly tapering to the bottom. Below the rim is inscribed with six characters reading "Da Ming Cheng Hua Nian Zhi" (made during Cheng Hua Period of the Ming Dynasty) in ink.

Collected by Zhang Yazong

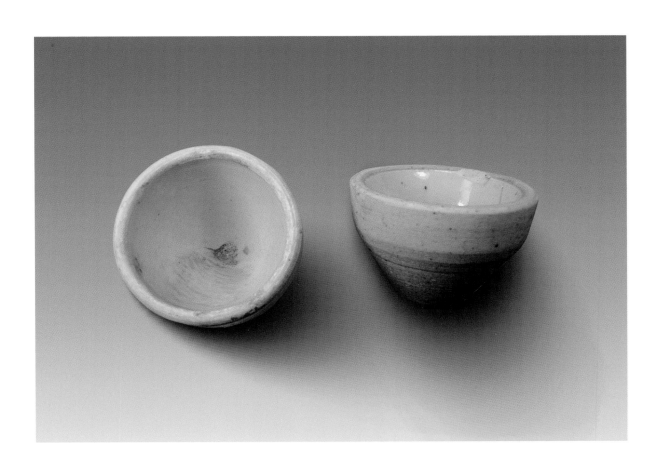

煎参汤杯

明

瓷质

口径 7 厘米，高 4.9 厘米

Ginseng Soup Slow-boiling Cups

Ming Dynasty

Porcelain

Mouth Diameter 7 cm/ Height 4.9 cm

2件。形似杯状，敞口，圆唇，折腹，下腹斜收，平底。厚胎。器身外侧半施白釉，底无釉。为煎参用汤锅。

张雅宗藏

The two cup-shaped pots have a flared mouth, a round rim, a folded belly tapering to the bottom, a flat bottom, and thick pottery body. The exterior except the bottom is covered with white glaze. The cup was used to slow boil ginseng soup.

Collected by Zhang Yazong

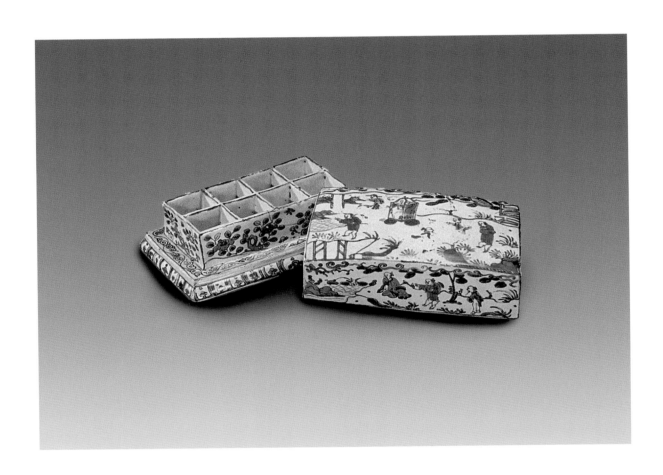

五彩多子盒

明

瓷质

长 22.4 厘米，宽 14 厘米，高 8.1 厘米

Multi-colored Box Set

Ming Dynasty

Porcelain

Length 22.4 cm/ Width 14 cm/ Height 8.1 cm

盒为大平底的长方形，内分为 8 个相同的小格，上有长槽形盖。在洁白的胎釉上，以红、绿、褐、黄、蓝多种颜色绘出周敦颐爱莲图、牡丹图和梅花图，底部有"大明万历年制"的题款。该藏品反映了明末五彩瓷器的特有风格。

首都博物馆藏

The oblong porcelain box has a flat bottom. It contains eight uniform compartments with a long groove-shaped lid. On the pure white glaze there are patterns of lotus, peony and plum blossoms which are decorated in red, green, brown, yellow, and blue. The bottom of the box is inscribed with six characters reading "Da Ming Wan Li Nian Zhi" (made during Wanli Period of the Ming Dynasty). The artifact reflects the special style of Multi-colored porcelain in the late Ming Dynasty.

Preserved in The Capital Museum

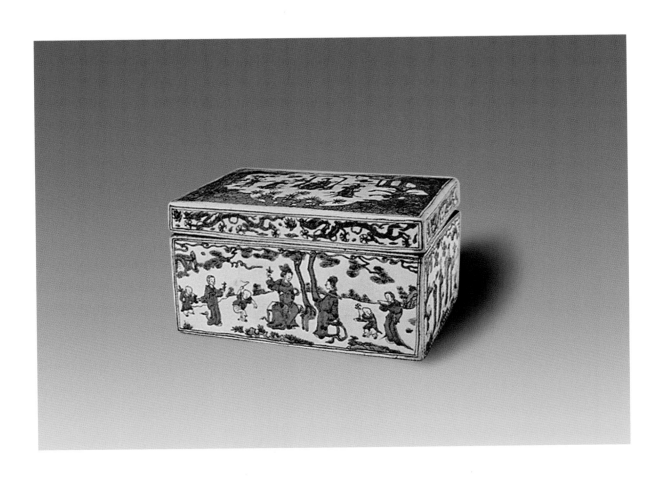

青花童戏图长方盒

明

瓷质

长 27.4 厘米，宽 16 厘米，高 16 厘米

Blue-and-white Oblong Box with Playing Children

Ming Dynasty

Porcelain

Length 27.4 cm/ Width 16 cm/ Height 16 cm

盒为长方形，造型浑厚。盖面及底之四壁均
绘童戏纹，包括斗草、鞭陀螺等。其中鞭陀
螺的儿童正弓腰甩鞭猛抽地上正在旋转的陀
螺，生活气息浓厚。

天津市艺术博物馆藏

The oblong porcelain box has a simple and
solemn modelling. The lid and the four walls
are decorated with children playing a revolving
top or the grass game. The child playing with
the top is bending over and whipping the
spinning top. The scene is full of vitality.
Preserved in Tianjin Art Museum

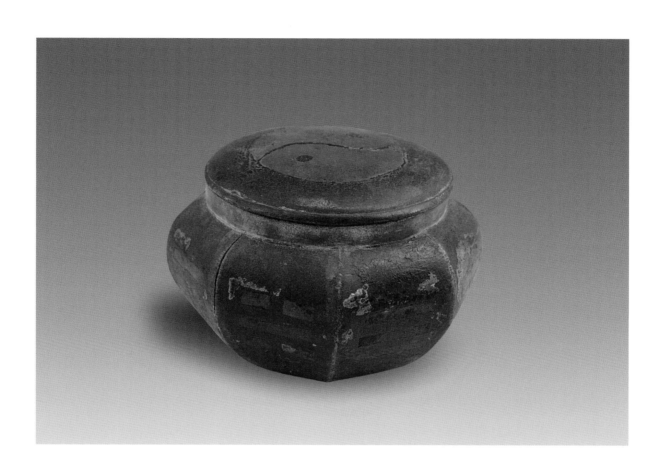

八卦纹药盒

明

瓷质

口径 12 厘米，高 12 厘米

Medicine Box with Eight Diagrams Motifs

Ming Dynasty

Porcelain

Mouth Diameter 12 cm/ Height 12 cm

直口，八棱瓜形腹，腹上八面分别刻有八卦
纹饰，配盖，盖上绘阴阳鱼纹。盛装中药器具。

北京御生堂中医药博物馆藏

The box has a vertical mouth and an octagonal
melon-shaped belly. The eight sides of the
belly are decorated with the patterns of Eight
Diagrams. The lid is painted with Yin and Yang
fish motifs. It was a tool for storing traditional
Chinese medicine.
Preserved in Chinese Medicine Museum of
Beijing Yu Sheng Tang Drugstore

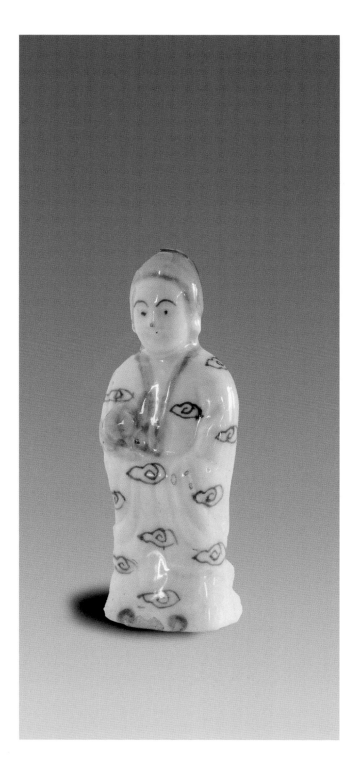

青花女瓷俑

明

瓷质

底长 5.5 厘米，底宽 4.5 厘米，高 15.2 厘米

Blue-and-white Female Figurine

Ming Dynasty

Porcelain

Bottom Length 5.5 cm/ Bottom Width 4.5 cm/

Height 15.2 cm

女子头裹巾帽，身穿开胸长衫，衣服衬以朵云纹，手托一朵含苞待放的荷花。形态文静、慈祥。全身施白釉，白釉莹润，微微闪青。底露胎，现淡淡火石红色。万历年间作品。

李牧之藏

The woman with a puggree wears an open gown decorated with cloud patterns and holds a budding lotus. Her facial expression is quiet and gracious. The whole body of the figurine is covered with white and mellow glaze with a glaucous tinge. The bottom, which is exposed without glaze, is light iron red. The figurine was made during Wanli Period of the Ming Dynasty. Collected by Li Muzhi

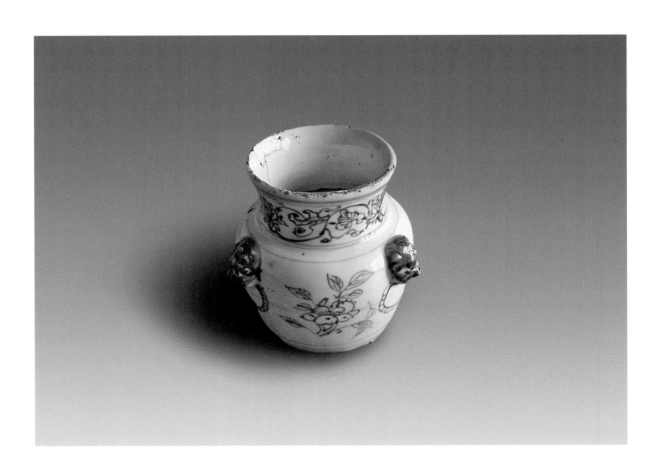

唾盂

明

瓷质

口径 6 厘米，高 8.5 厘米

Spittoon

Ming Dynasty

Porcelain

Mouth Diameter 6 cm/ Height 8.5 cm

敞口，高颈，腹微鼓，圈足，肩部贴塑三个
铺首纹。器表饰青花花卉纹，釉色莹润，青
花色泽鲜明，造型规整。四川文物商店征集。

成都中医药大学中医药传统文化博物馆藏

The spittoon has a flared mouth, a long neck,
a slightly bulged belly, and a ring foot. Three
animal heads are pasted on the shoulder. Its
surface is decorated with blue-and-white
flowers and plants. The color of the glaze is
mellow and bright. The shape of the spittoon
is regular. The artifact was collected from an
antique shop in Sichuan Province.

Preserved in Museum of Traditional Chinese
Medicine Culture, Chengdu University of
Traditional Chinese Medicine

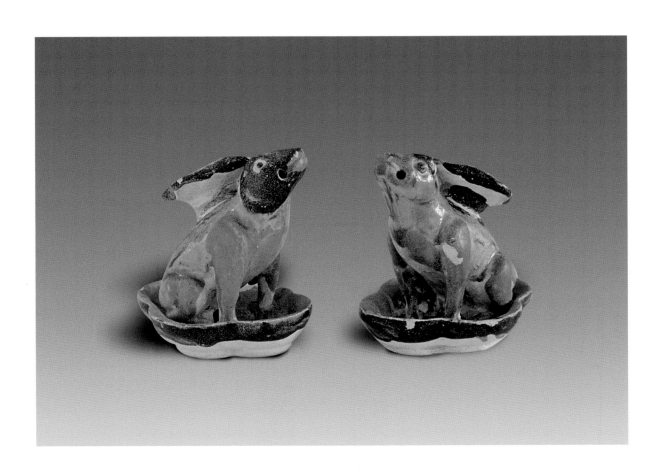

三彩蛙形灯

明

瓷质

高 10 厘米

Tri-colored Frog-shaped Lamps

Ming Dynasty

Porcelain

Height 10 cm

整个灯形像一个活的青蛙立于荷塘中的荷叶上，蛙首上扬，仰望长空。器底是一个盛油的荷叶形盏托，蛙背有一个加油用的荷叶形漏斗，蛙腹中空。漏斗、蛙腹与盏托相通，蛙嘴两角各有一个圆孔，用于放灯芯。灰白胎，施化妆土，釉色有黄色、青绿色和茶褐色，釉层开细碎冰片。为出土明器。

吴德蔚藏

Each lamp is shaped like a living frog with a hollow abdomen, which is standing on a lotus leaf in a pond, looking up into the sky. The base of the lamp is a lotus-shaped tray which serves as oil container. On the back of the lamps there is a lotus-shaped funnel. The funnel, the frog's abdomen and the tray are interlinked with each other. On both corners of the frog's mouth there are two tiny holes used for placing the wicks in. The lamps have grayish white pottery body coated with engobe. The glaze consists of such colors as yellow, green and brown with fine crackles. The lamps were burial items.
Collected by Wu Dewei

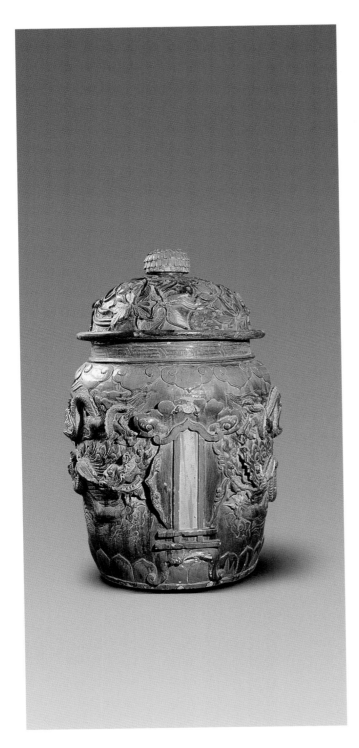

黄绿釉蟠龙瓷棺

明

瓷质

腹径 84 厘米，高 132 厘米

Yellowish Green-glazed Urn Coffin with Coiled Dragons

Ming Dynasty

Porcelain

Belly Diameter 84 cm/ Height 132 cm

短颈，丰肩，鼓腹，腹以下内收，盖饰宝珠
形纽，与棺身子母扣合。周身雕刻花纹，腹
上部为一周如意纹，近底部为仰莲瓣纹，腹
部饰龙穿牡丹纹。通体施黄绿釉，纹饰精细，
釉色匀称光亮。此棺器型硕大，气势雄伟，
雕饰奇巧，釉色鲜艳，流光夺目，为明代琉
璃器中的杰出代表作。

山西博物院藏

The coffin has a short neck, a plump shoulder,
and a bulged and tapered belly. The lid is
decorated with a pearl-shaped knob. The whole
body is carved with patterns. The upper part
of the belly is decorated with a circle of Ruyi
patterns and the lower part is decorated with
lotus petal patterns. The belly is patterned with
delicate dragons and peonies. The whole body is
decorated with yellowish-green glaze which is
lustrous and even. The huge coffin is imposing
with ingenious carving and brilliant glaze. It
is indeed a masterpiece of colored glaze of the
Ming Dynasty.

Preserved in Shanxi Museum

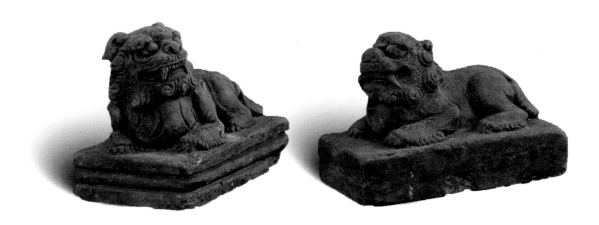

狮镇

明

陶质

长 17.8 厘米，宽 9.5 厘米，高 12 厘米，重 1500 克

狮镇一对。长方形底座，底座上为一形态逼真的雄卧狮。完整无损。

陕西医史博物馆藏

Lion-shasped Paperweight

Ming Dynasty

Pottery

Length 17.8 cm/ Width 9.5 cm/ Height 12 cm/ Weight 1,500 g

The pair lively male lions are crouching on a rectangular base. It is in good condition.

Preserved in Shaanxi Museum of Medical History

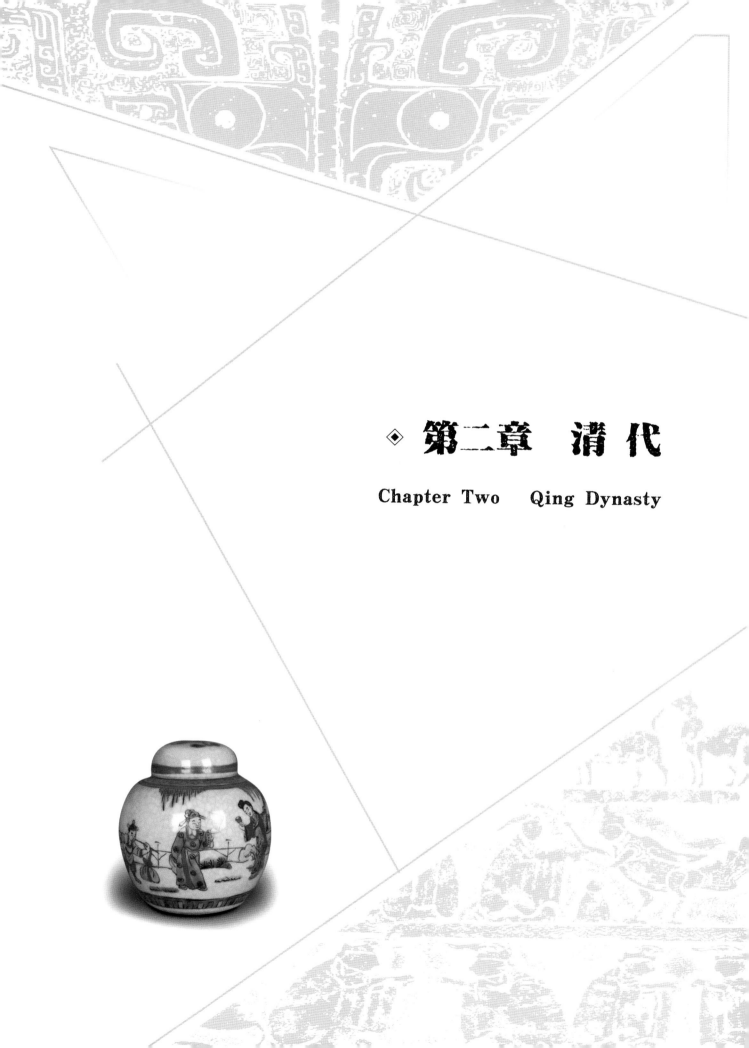

◈ 第二章　清　代

Chapter Two　Qing Dynasty

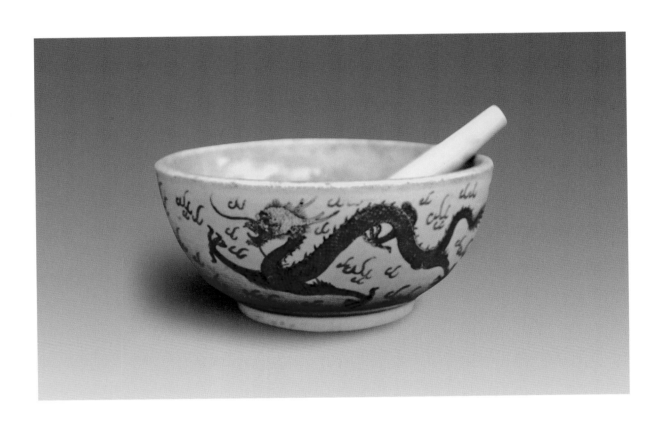

矾红色龙纹擂钵及杵

清

瓷质

杵：长 12.06 厘米，重 98 克

钵：口外径 16.18 厘米，底径 9.07 厘米，深 6.4 厘米，重 710 克

Orangish Red Dragon-patterned Mortar and Pestle

Qing Dynasty

Porcelain

Pestle: Length 12.06 cm/ Weight 98 g

Mortar: Mouth Outer Diameter 16.18 cm/ Bottom Diameter 9.07 cm/ Depth 6.4 cm/ Weight 710 g

杵呈棒状，钵为敞口，平底，圈足，表面绘釉里红龙纹图案。用于加工炮制药物。

广东中医药博物馆藏

The pestle is shaped like a stick. The mortar has a flared mouth, a flat bottom, and a ring foot. The outer wall is painted with red dragon patterns. The collection was used for processing and preparing medicine.

Preserved in Guangdong Chinese Medicine Museum

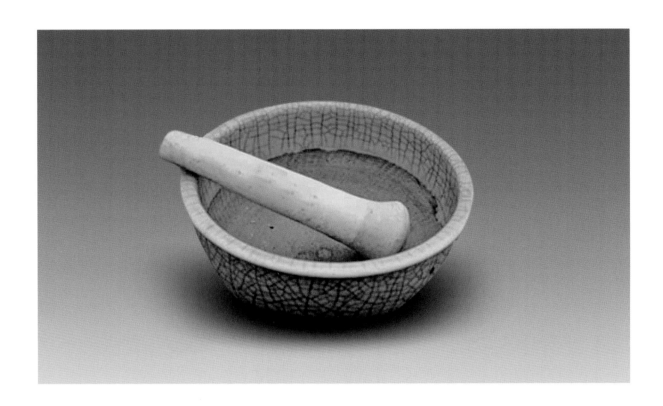

仿哥窑大擂钵及杵

清

瓷质

杵：长 21 厘米，重 510 克

钵：口外径 24 厘米，底径 13.5 厘米，深 9.5 厘米，重 2200 克

Mortar and Pestle Imitating Ge Kiln

Qing Dynasty

Porcelain

Pestle: Length 21 cm/ Weight 510 g

Mortar: Mouth Outer Diameter 24 cm/ Bottom Diameter 13.5 cm/ Depth 9.5 cm/ Weight 2,200 g

杵呈棒状。钵为敞口，平底，圈足，器表有
仿哥窑的开片。用于加工炮制药物。

广东中医药博物馆藏

The pestle is shaped like a stick. The mortar
has a flared mouth, a flat bottom, and a ring
foot. On the surface there are some imitated
Ge Kiln's crackles. The collection was used for
processing and preparing medicinal ingredients.
Preserved in Guangdong Chinese Medicine Museum

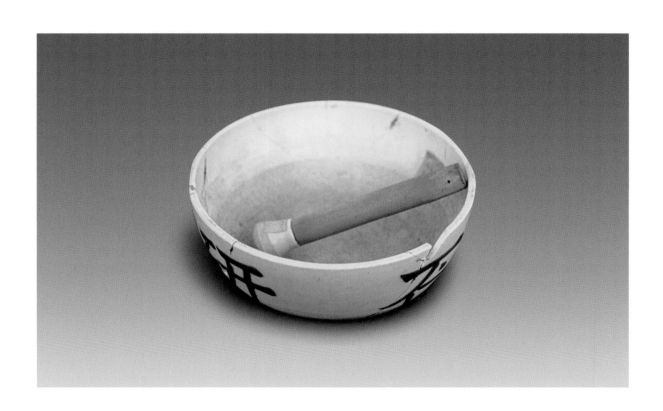

金鸡石瓷大擂钵及杵

清

瓷质

杵：长 16.7 厘米，头径 3.55 厘米，柄径 2.5 厘米，重 56 克

钵：口外径 20.8 厘米，底径 11 厘米，通高 10.4 厘米，重 1244 克

Golden Rooster Rock and Porcelain Mortar and Pestle

Qing Dynasty

Porcelain

Pestle: Length 16.7 cm/ Head Diameter 3.55 cm/ Handle Diameter 2.5 cm/ Weight 56 g

Mortar: Mouth Outer Diameter 20.8 cm/ Bottom Diameter 11 cm/ Height 10.4 cm/ Weight 1,244 g

杵呈棒状，瓷质杵头，木质杵柄。钵形似碗，敞口，平底，通体施白釉，器表上书有"研石捣金"四字。用于加工炮制药物。

广东中医药博物馆藏

The porcelain pestle is shaped like a stick with a wooden handle. The mortar is shaped like a bowl with a flared mouth and a flat bottom. The pottery body is coated with white glaze. On the surface there are four Chinese characters reading "Yan Shi Dao Jin" indicating the function of the mortar. The collection was utilized for processing and preparing medicinal ingredients.

Preserved in Guangdong Chinese Medicine Museum

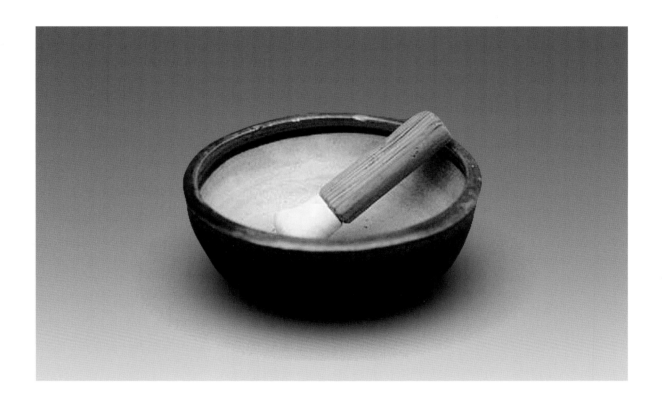

黑釉擂钵及杵

清

瓷质

杵：重 68 克

钵：口外径 18.3 厘米，底径 9 厘米，通高 7.5 厘米，深 7.1 厘米，重 750 克

Black Glazed Mortar and Pestle

Qing Dynasty

Porcelain

Pestle: Weight 68 g

Mortar: Mouth Outer Diameter 18.3 cm/ Bottom Diameter 9 cm/ Height 7.5 cm/ Depth 7.1 cm/ Weight 750 g

杵为白色瓷杵头，木质杵柄。钵为敞口，平底。
黑釉瓷质，用于炮制加工药物。

广东中医药博物馆藏

The pestle, which is made of white porcelain,
has a wooden handle. The porcelain mortar
is shaped like a bowl with a flared mouth and
a flat bottom. It is coated with black glaze.
The collection was utilized for processing and
preparing medicine.

Preserved in Guangdong Chinese Medicine Museum

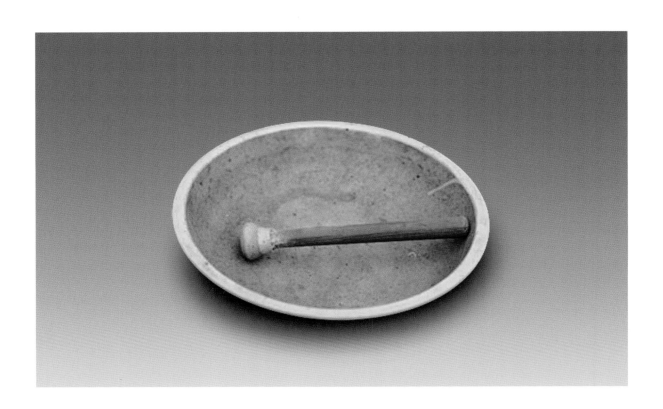

白釉钵及杵

清

瓷质

杵：长 16.64 厘米，重 27 克

钵：口外径 22.6 厘米，底径 13.8 厘米，深 6.2 厘米，重 955 克

White-glazed Mortar and Pestle

Qing Dynasty

Porcelain

Pestle: Length 16.64 cm/ Weight 27 g

Mortar: Mouth Outer Diameter 22.6 cm/ Bottom Diameter 13.8 cm/ Depth 6.2 cm/ Weight 955 g

杵呈棒状，瓷质杵头，木质杵柄。钵敞口，
宽沿，小平底，通体施白釉。用于加工炮制
药物。

广东中医药博物馆藏

The porcelain pestle is shaped like a stick with a
wooden handle. The mortar has a flared mouth,
a wide rim, and a small flat bottom. The body
is coated with white glaze. The collection was
utilized for processing and preparing medicine.

Preserved in Guangdong Chinese Medicine Museum

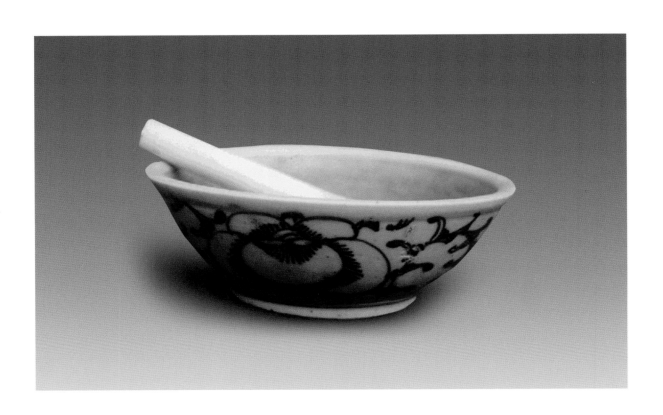

青花擂钵及杵一套七件之一

清

瓷质

杵：长 14.3 厘米，重 115 克

钵：口外径 17.38 厘米， 底径 9.48 厘米， 深 5.75 厘米，重 460 克

Seven Blue-and-white Mortars and Pestles（ Ⅰ ）

Qing Dynasty

Porcelain

Pestle: Length 14.3 cm/ Weight 115 g

Mortar: Mouth Outer Diameter 17.38 cm/ Bottom Diameter 9.48 cm/ Depth 5.75 cm/ Weight 460 g

杵呈棒状。钵为敞口，平底，圈足，器表饰
青花图案。用于加工炮制药物。

广东中医药博物馆藏

The pestle is shaped like a stick. The mortar has
a flared mouth, a flat bottom, and a ring foot. It
is decorated with white-and-blue patterns on the
surface. The collection was used for processing
and preparing medicine.

Preserved in Guangdong Chinese Medicine Museum

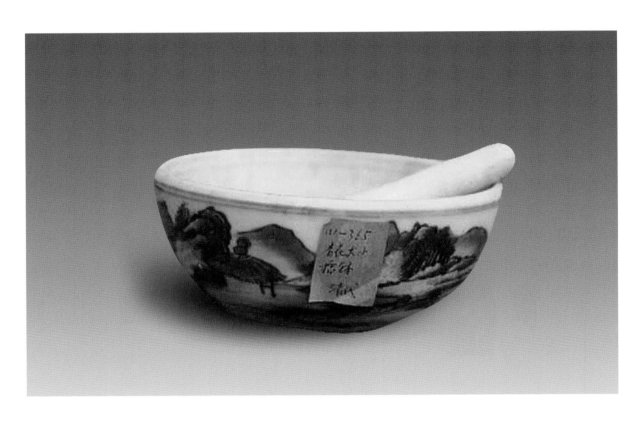

青花擂钵及杵一套七件之二

清

瓷质

杵：长 11 厘米，重 102 克

钵：口外径 14.96 厘米，底径 6.84 厘米，深 5.5 厘米，重 650 克

Seven Blue-and-white Mortars and Pestles（Ⅱ）

Qing Dynasty

Porcelain

Pestle: Length 11 cm/ Weight 102 g

Mortar: Mouth Outer Diameter 14.96 cm/ Bottom Diameter 6.84 cm/ Depth 5.5 cm/ Weight 650 g

杵呈棒状。钵为敞口，平底，器表饰青花山
水图案。用于加工炮制药物。

广东中医药博物馆藏

The pestle is shaped like a stick. The mortar has
a flared mouth and a flat bottom. It is decorated
with white-and-blue landscape on the surface.
The collection was used for processing and
preparing medicine.

Preserved in Guangdong Chinese Medicine Museum

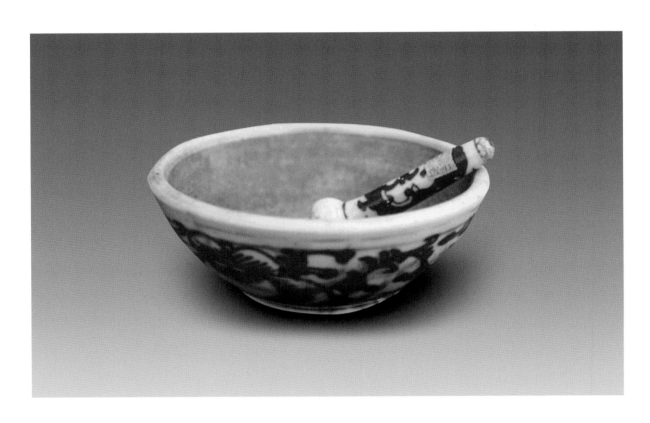

青花擂钵及杵一套七件之三

清

瓷质

杵：长 8.37 厘米，重 41 克

钵：口外径 13.09 厘米，底径 7.44 厘米，深 5.1 厘米，重 305 克

Seven Blue-and-white Mortars and Pestles（Ⅲ）

Qing Dynasty

Porcelain

Pestle: Length 8.37 cm/ Weight 41 g

Mortar: Mouth Outer Diameter 13.09 cm/ Bottom Diameter 7.44 cm/ Depth 5.1 cm/ Weight 305 g

杵呈棒状。钵为敞口，平底，圈足，器表饰
青花图案。用于加工炮制药物。

广东中医药博物馆藏

The pestle is stick-shaped. The mortar has
a flared rim, a flat bottom, and a ring foot.
Its surface is decorated with blue-and-white
flower patterns. The collection was utilized for
processing and preparing medicinal ingredients.
Preserved in Guangdong Chinese Medicine Museum

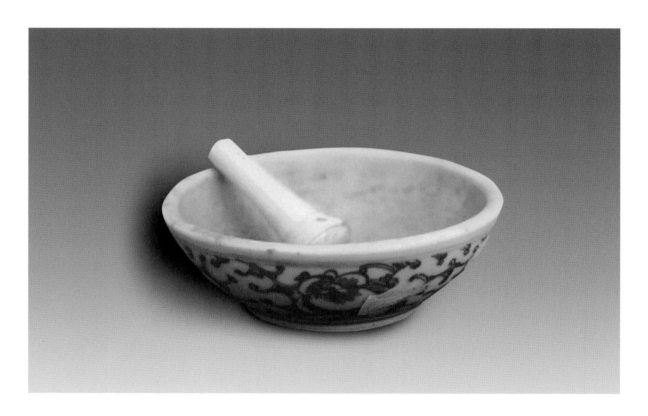

青花擂钵及杵一套七件之四

清

瓷质

杵：长 7.39 厘米，重 38 克

钵：口外径 13.33 厘米，底径 7.85 厘米，深 4.3 厘米，钵重 305 克

Seven Blue-and-white Mortars and Pestles（Ⅳ）

Qing Dynasty

Porcelain

Pestle: Length 7.39 cm/ Weight 38 g

Mortar: Mouth Outer Diameter 13.33 cm/ Bottom Diameter 7.85 cm/ Depth 4.3 cm/ Weight 305 g

杵呈棒状。钵为敞口，平底，圈足，器表饰
青花草木图案。用于加工炮制药物。

广东中医药博物馆藏

The pestle is stick-shaped. The mortar has
a flared rim, a flat bottom, and a ring foot.
Its surface is decorated with blue-and-white
flower and grass patterns. The collection was
utilized for processing and preparing medicinal
ingredients.

Preserved in Guangdong Chinese Medicine Museum

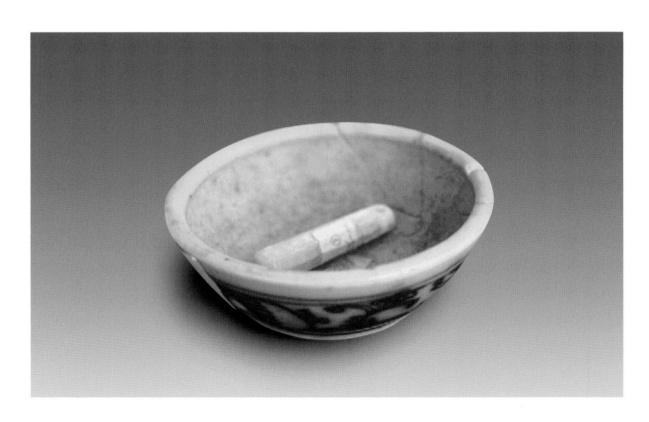

青花擂钵及杵一套七件之五

清

瓷质

杵：长 6.08 厘米，重 12 克

钵：口外径 10.64 厘米，底径 6.63 厘米，深 3.6 厘米，重 165 克

Seven Blue-and-white Mortars and Pestles（Ⅴ）

Qing Dynasty

Porcelain

Pestle: Length 6.08 cm/ Weight 12 g

Mortar: Mouth Outer Diameter 10.64 cm/ Bottom Diameter 6.63 cm/ Depth 3.6 cm/ Weight 165 g

杵呈棒状。钵为敞口，平底，器表饰青花图案。
用于加工炮制药物。

广东中医药博物馆藏

The pestle is stick-shaped. The mortar has a
flared rim and a flat bottom. The surface is
decorated with blue-and-white flower patterns.
The collection was utilized for processing and
preparing medicinal ingredients.

Preserved in Guangdong Chinese Medicine Museum

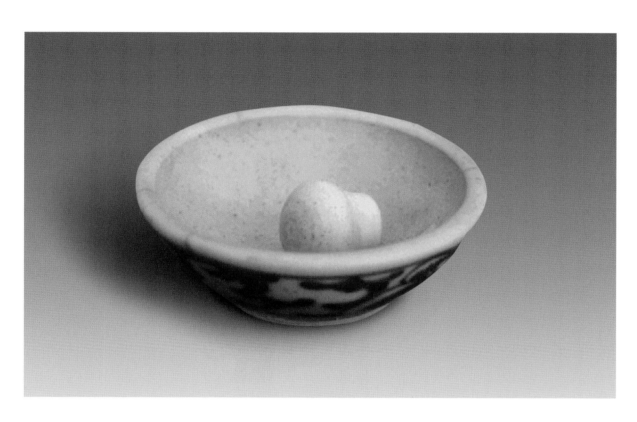

青花擂钵及杵一套七件之六

清

瓷质

杵：长 2.85 厘米，重 24 克

钵：口外径 10.38 厘米，底径 6.21 厘米，深 3.7 厘米，重 150 克

Seven Blue-and-white Mortars and Pestles（Ⅵ）

Qing Dynasty

Porcelain

Pestle: Length 2.85 cm/ Weight 24 g

Mortar: Mouth Outer Diameter 10.38 cm/ Bottom Diameter 6.21 cm/ Depth 3.7 cm/ Weight 150 g

杵呈棒状。钵为敞口，平底，圈足，器表饰
青花图案。用于加工炮制药物。

广东中医药博物馆藏

The pestle is stick-shaped. The mortar has
a flared rim, a flat bottom, and a ring foot.
The surface is decorated with blue-and-white
flower patterns. The collection was utilized for
processing and preparing medicinal ingredients.
Preserved in Guangdong Chinese Medicine Museum

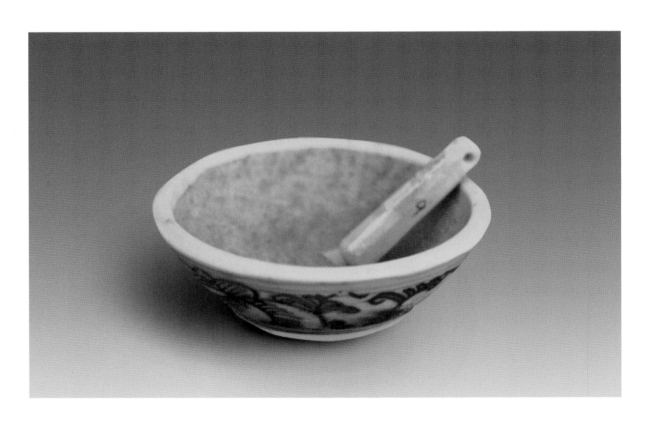

青花擂钵及杵一套七件之七

清

瓷质

杵：长 6.08 厘米，重 12 克

钵：口外径 10.12 厘米，底径 6.15 厘米，深 3.2 厘米，重 130 克

Seven Blue-and-white Mortars and Pestles（Ⅶ）

Qing Dynasty

Porcelain

Pestle: Length 6.08 cm/ Weight 12 g

Mortar: Mouth Outer Diameter 10.12 cm/ Bottom Diameter 6.15 cm/ Depth 3.2 cm/ Weight 130 g

杵呈棒状。钵为敞口，平底，圈足，器表饰
青花图案。用于加工炮制药物。

广东中医药博物馆藏

The pestle is stick-shaped. The mortar has
a flared rim, a flat bottom, and a ring foot.
Its surface is decorated with blue-and-white
flower patterns. The collection was utilized for
processing medicinal ingredients.
Preserved in Guangdong Chinese Medicine Museum

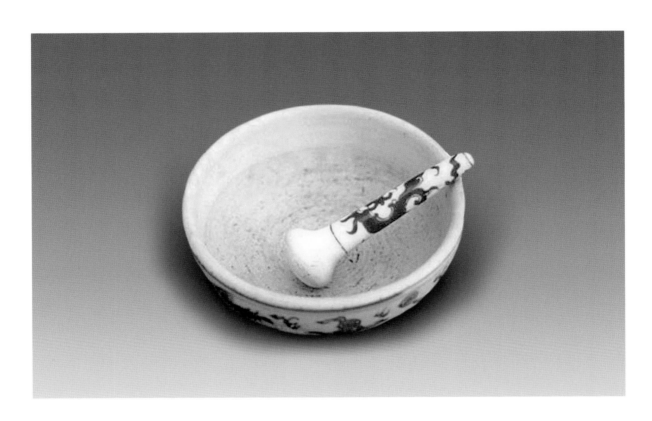

青花擂钵及杵

清

瓷质

杵：长 9.36 厘米，重 47.5 克

钵：口外径 12.6 厘米，底径 7.11 厘米，通高 5.2 厘米，深 3.8 厘米，重 345 克

Blue-and-white Mortar and Pestle

Qing Dynasty

Porcelain

Pestle: Length 9.36 cm/ Weight 47.5 g

Mortar: Mouth Outer Diameter 12.6 cm/ Bottom Diameter 7.11 cm/ Height 5.2 cm/ Depth 3.8 cm/ Weight 345 g

杵呈棒状。钵为敞口，平底，器表饰青花图案。
用于捣碎药物。

广东中医药博物馆藏

The pestle is stick-shaped. The mortar has
a flared rim and a flat bottom. Its surface is
decorated with blue-and-white flower patterns.
The collection was utilized for mashing
medicinal ingredients.

Preserved in Guangdong Chinese Medicine Museum

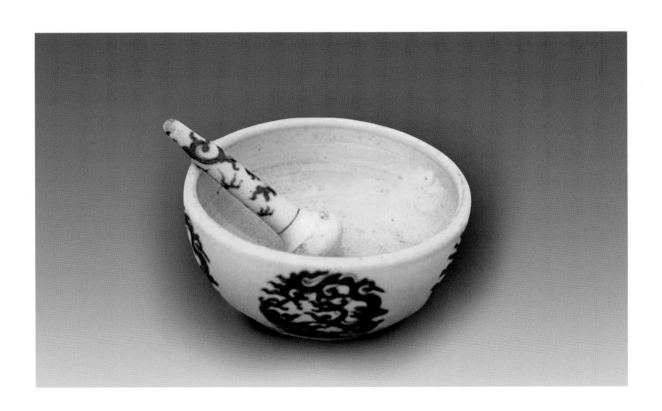

青花擂钵及杵

清

瓷质

杵：长 9.45 厘米，重 47.2 克

钵：口外径 12.61 厘米，底径 8.47 厘米，通高 6.17 厘米，深 4.5 厘米，重 410 克

Blue-and-white Mortar and Pestle

Qing Dynasty

Porcelain

Pestle: Length 9.45 cm/ Weight 47.2 g

Mortar: Mouth Outer Diameter 12.61 cm/ Bottom Diameter 8.47 cm/ Height 6.17 cm/ Depth 4.5 cm/ Weight 410 g

杵呈棒状。钵为敞口，平底，器表饰青花图案。
用于捣碎研细药物。

广东中医药博物馆藏

The pestle is stick-shaped. The mortar has a flared rim and a flat bottom. Its surface is decorated with blue-and-white flower patterns. The collection was utilized for mashing and porphyrizing medicinal ingredients.

Preserved in Guangdong Chinese Medicine Museum

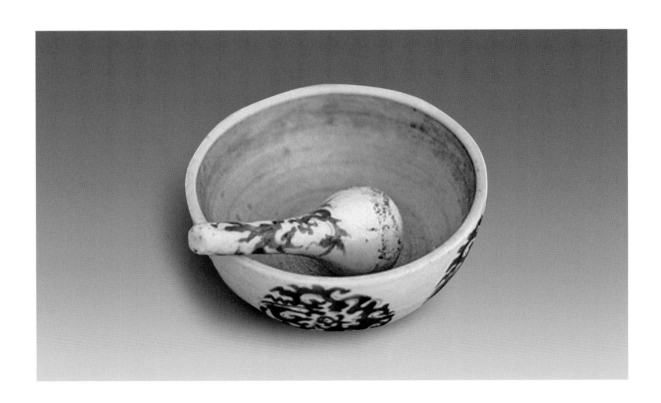

青花擂钵带杵

清

瓷质

杵：重 127 克

钵：外口径 13.8 厘米，底口径 9.3 厘米，通高 6.3 厘米，腹深 5.48 厘米，重 438 克

Blue-and-white Mortar and Pestle

Qing Dynasty

Porcelain

Pestle: Weight 127 g

Mortar: Mouth Outer Diameter 13.8 cm/ Bottom Diameter 9.3 cm/ Height 6.3 cm/ Belly Depth 5.48 cm/ Weight 438 g

杵呈棒状。钵为敞口，平底，器表饰青花图案。
用于捣碎研细药物。

广东中医药博物馆藏

The pestle is stick-shaped. The mortar has
a flared rim and a flat bottom. Its surface is
decorated with blue-and-white flower patterns.
The collection was utilized for mashing and
porphyrizing medicinal ingredients.

Preserved in Guangdong Chinese Medicine Museum

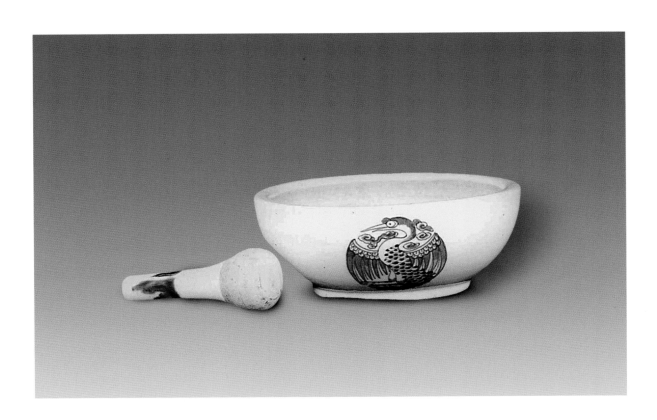

青花研钵及杵

清

瓷质

杵：长 18 厘米

钵：底径 5 厘米，高 13 厘米

Blue-and-white Mortar and Pestle

Qing Dynasty

Porcelain

Pestle: Length 18 cm

Mortar: Bottom Diameter 5 cm/ Height 13 cm

杵呈棒状。钵为敞口，平底，圈足，器表绘
青花团鹤纹图案。研药器具。

上海中医药博物馆藏

The pestle is stick-shaped. The mortar has a
flared mouth, a flat bottom, and a ring foot.
Its surface is painted with blue-and-white
crane patterns. The mortar was utilized for
porphyrizing medicinal ingredients.
Preserved in Shanghai Museum of Traditional
Chinese Medicine

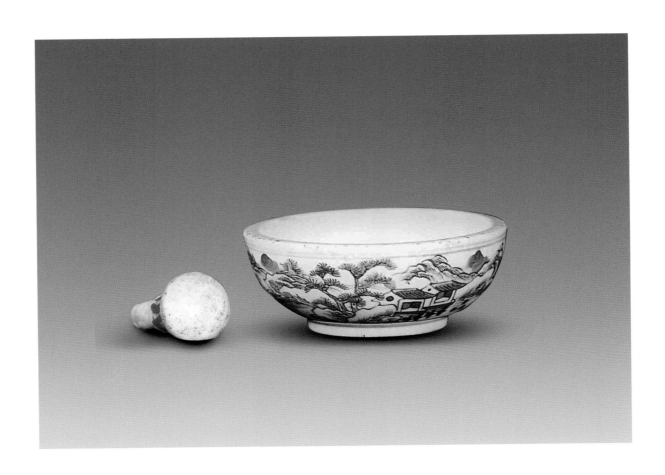

青花研钵及杵

清

瓷质

口径 8.5 厘米，底径 4.5 厘米，高 4 厘米

Blue-and-white Mortar and Pestle

Qing Dynasty

Porcelain

Mouth Diameter 8.5 cm/ Bottom Diameter 4.5 cm/ Height 4 cm

敞口，平底，圈足，带一瓷质杵。器表绘青
花山水图案。研药器具。

上海中医药博物馆藏

The mortar has a flared mouth, a flat bottom,
and a ring foot. Its surface is painted with blue-
and-white landscape patterns. A porcelain
pestle goes with the mortar. The collection was
utilized for porphyrizing medicinal ingredients.
Preserved in Shanghai Museum of Traditional
Chinese Medicine

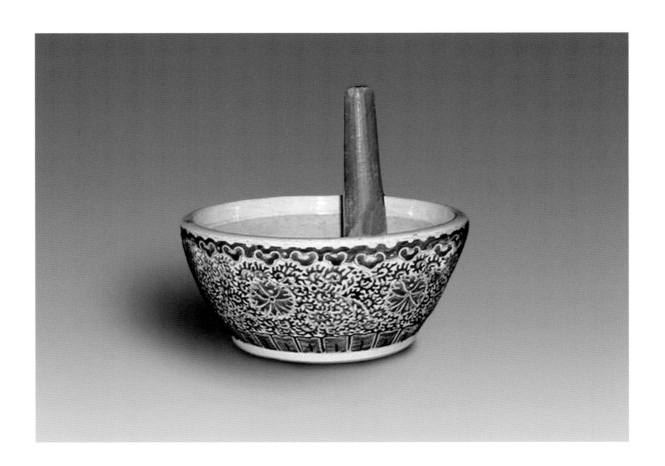

青花瓷研钵

清

瓷质

口径 27.5 厘米，底径 12.5 厘米，通高 18 厘米，重 3650 克

Blue-and-white Porcelain Mortar

Qing Dynasty

Porcelain

Mouth Diameter 27.5 cm/ Bottom Diameter 12.5 cm/ Height 18 cm/ Weight 3,650 g

直口，斜腹，圈足。口沿处一圈云纹，腹为
缠枝纹，带一杵。研药器具。江苏扬州征集。

陕西医史博物馆藏

The mortar has a vertical mouth, an inclined
belly, and a ring foot. Its mouth rim is decorated
with a circle of cloud patterns and its belly is
decorated with intertwining branch patterns.
The mortar goes with a pestle. The collection
was utilized for porphyrizing medicinal
ingredients. It was collected in Yangzhou City,
Jiangsu Province.

Preserved in Shaanxi Museum of Medical History

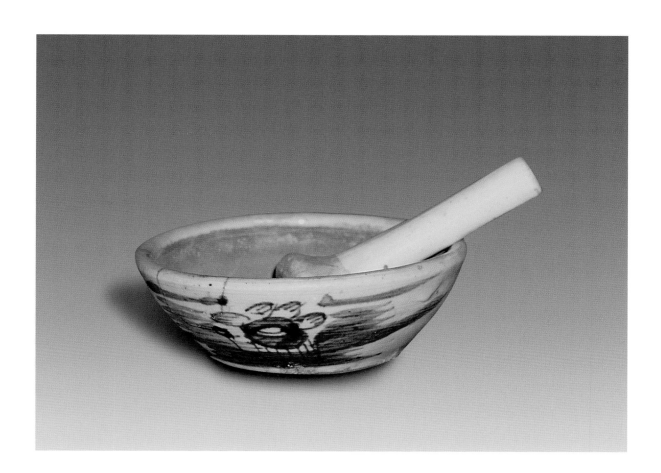

瓷研钵

清

瓷质

口径 13 厘米，底径 4 厘米，通高 8 厘米，重 350 克

Porcelain Mortar

Qing Dynasty

Porcelain

Mouth Diameter 13 cm/ Bottom Diameter 4 cm/ Height 8 cm/ Weight 350 g

敞口，斜腹，平底，带一瓷质杵。器表绘青
花图案。研药器具。陕西汉中征集。

陕西医史博物馆藏

The mortar has a flared mouth, an inclined
belly, and a flat bottom. Its surface is decorated
with blue-and-white flower patterns. A porcelain
pestle goes with the mortar. The collection was
utilized for porphyrizing medicinal ingredients.
It was collected in Hanzhong City, Shaanxi
Province.

Preserved in Shaanxi Museum of Medical History

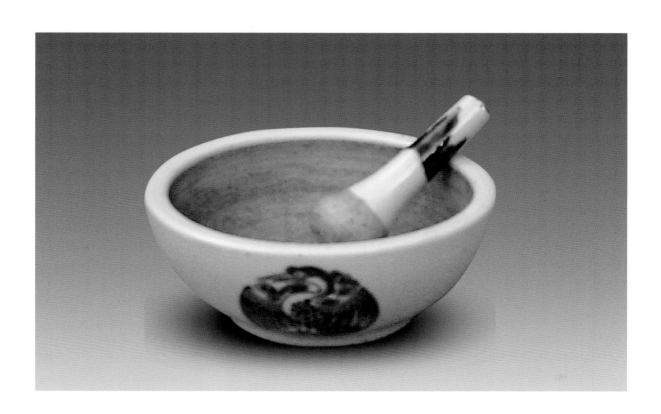

青花研钵

清

瓷质

杵：长 8 厘米

钵：口外径 12.9 厘米，底径 7 厘米，通高 5.2 厘米

Blue-and-white Mortar

Qing Dynasty

Porcelain

Pestle: Length 8 cm

Mortar: Mouth Outer Diameter 12.9 cm/ Bottom Diameter 7 cm/ Height 5.2 cm

杵呈棒状。钵为敞口，平底，圈足。器表绘
青花图案。制药用具。

中华医学会 / 上海中医药大学医史博物

The pestle is shaped like a stick. The mortar
has a flared mouth, a flat bottom, and a ring
foot. Its surface is decorated with blue-and-
white patterns. The collection was utilized for
preparing medicine.
Preserved in Chinese Medical Association/
Museum of Chinese Medicine, Shanghai
University of Traditional Chinese Medicine

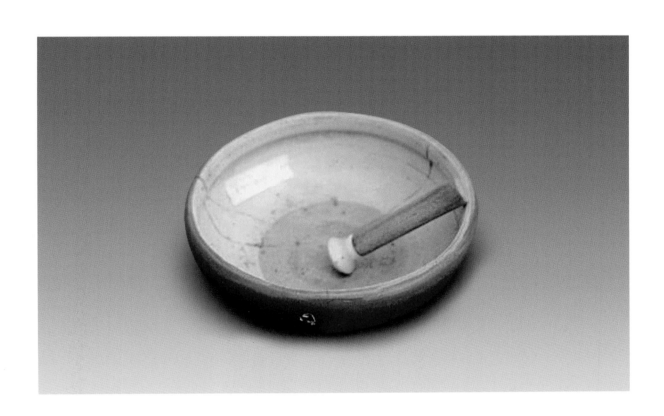

祭蓝瓷钵

清

瓷质

杵：长 11.3 厘米，重 31 克

钵：口外径 20.2 厘米，底径 10.7 厘米，通高 8.3 厘米，重 105 克

Sacrificial Blue-glazed Mortar

Qing Dynasty

Porcelain

Pestle: Length 11.3 cm/ Weight 31 g

Mortar: Mouth Outer Diameter 20.2 cm/ Bottom Diameter 10.7 cm/ Height 8.3 cm/ Weight 105 g

杵呈棒状，木柄瓷头。钵体形似盒，平底，近底处有三只假足。白胎，内施白釉，外施蓝釉。研细药物用。

广东中医药博物馆藏

The porcelain pestle is shaped like a stick with a wooden handle. The mortar is shaped like a box, with a flat bottom and three feet near the bottom. It has a white pottery body coated with white glaze inside and blue glaze outside. The collection was utilized for porphyrizing drug ingredients.

Preserved in Guangdong Chinese Medicine Museum

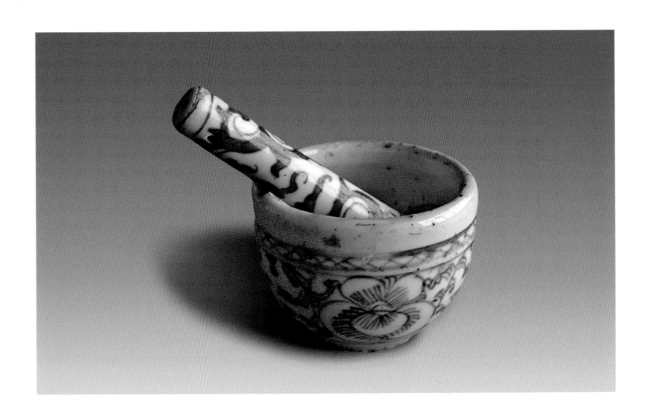

药臼

清

瓷质

杵：长11厘米

钵：口径8厘米，高6厘米

Medicine Mortar

Qing Dynasty

Porcelain

Pestle: Length 11 cm

Mortar: Mouth Diameter 8 cm/ Height 6 cm

敞口，直腹，下部内收，平底。外壁有青花
枝叶纹图案。研药器具。民间征集。

成都中医药大学中医药传统文化博物馆藏

The mortar has a flared mouth, a vertical and
tapered belly, and a flat bottom. Its wall is
decorated with blue-and-white branch and
leaf patterns. The mortar was utilized for
porphyrizing medicinal ingredients. It was
collected from a private owner.

Preserved in Museum of Traditional Chinese
Medicine Culture, Chengdu University of
Traditional Chinese Medicine

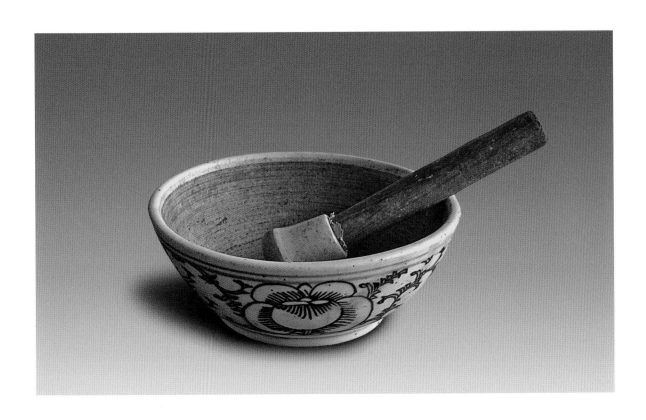

药臼

清

瓷质

杵：长 17 厘米

钵：口径 17.5 厘米，高 7 厘米

Medicine Mortar

Qing Dynasty

Porcelain

Pestle: Length 17 cm

Mortar: Mouth Diameter 17.5 cm/ Height 7 cm

敞口，腹内收，平底。腹部有青花缠枝纹饰。

研药器具。民间征集。

成都中医药大学中医药传统文化博物馆藏

The mortar has a flared mouth, a contracted belly, and a flat bottom. The belly is decorated with blue-and-white intertwining branch patterns. The mortar was utilized for porphyrizing medicinal ingredients. It was collected from a private owner. Preserved in Museum of Traditional Chinese Medicine Culture, Chengdu University of Traditional Chinese Medicine

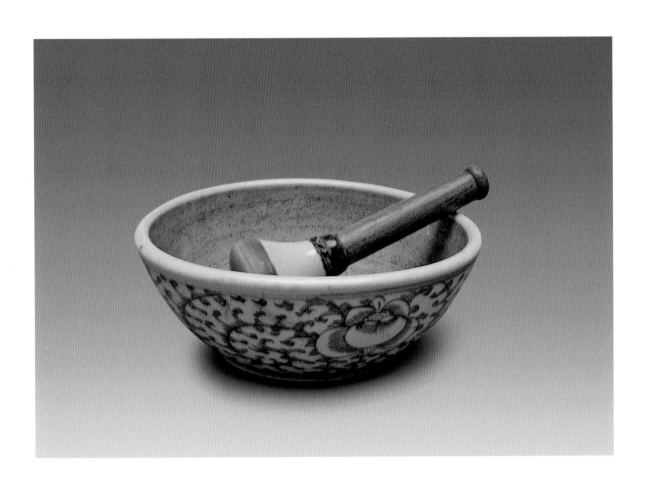

乳钵

清

瓷质

高 7.5 厘米

Mortar

Qing Dynasty

Porcelain

Height 7.5 cm

敞口，腹内收，平底，带杵。外壁饰青花缠枝纹。研药器具。四川省文物商店征集。

成都中医药大学中医药传统文化博物馆藏

The mortar has a flared mouth, a contracted belly and a flat bottom. Its wall is decorated with blue-and-white intertwining branch patterns. There is a pestle that goes with it. The mortar was utilized for porphyrizing medicinal ingredients. It was collected from a cultural relics shop in Sichuan Province.

Preserved in Museum of Traditional Chinese Medicine Culture, Chengdu University of Traditional Chinese Medicine

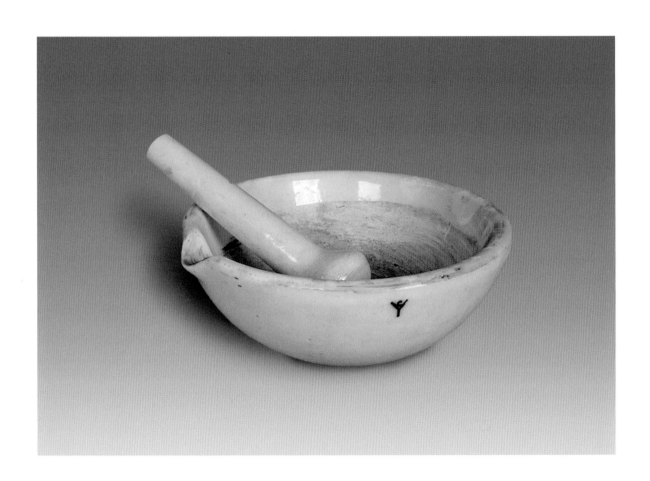

研钵

清

瓷质

口内径 21 厘米，口外径 24.6 厘米，高 8.9 厘米

Mortar

Qing Dynasty

Porcelain

Mouth Inner Diameter 21 cm/ Mouth Outer Diameter 24.6 cm/ Height 8.9 cm

敞口，平底，一端有流，嘴略弯曲，肩部有两系四孔，配瓷杵。通身施白釉，内面露土褐色胎，钵口外侧一处标青花字母"CY"组成图案，底无款。制药工具。1955 年入藏。

中华医学会／上海中医药大学医史博物馆藏

The mortar has a flared mouth and a flat bottom. On one side of the rim there is a spout with a slightly curved mouth. There are two handles and four holes on the shoulder. A porcelain pestle goes with the mortar. The mortar is coated with white glaze while the interior has a drab pottery body. On the outside of its rim there are patterns made up of blue-and-white letters "CY". There is no inscription on the bottom. The mortar was utilized for preparing medicine. It was collected by the museum in 1955.

Preserved in Chinese Medical Association/ Museum of Chinese Medicine, Shanghai University of Traditional Chinese Medicine

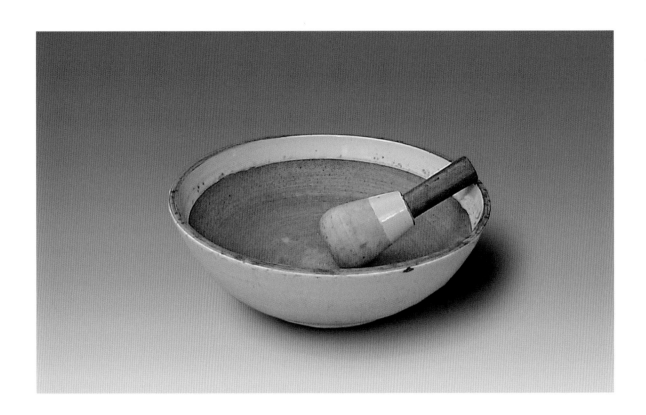

研钵

清

瓷质

杵：长 30.6 厘米，径 9.3 厘米

钵：口径 46 厘米，通高 15.2 厘米

Mortar

Qing Dynasty

Porcelain

Pestle: Length 30.6 cm/ Diameter 9.3 cm

Mortar: Mouth Diameter 46 cm/ Height 15.2 cm

杵为瓷杵头镶木柄。钵为平底，敞口，内面有旋纹和使用痕迹。白釉，口沿棕黄釉，工艺较好，体料厚重，便于研磨。制药工具。1957 年入藏。

中华医学会 / 上海中医药大学医史博物馆藏

The pestle has a porcelain head and a wooden handle. The mortar has a flared mouth and a flat bottom. The body is coated with white glaze while the rim is coated with yellow glaze. There are spiral patterns and traces of use on the inner wall. The collection has fine workmanship and is made of heavy and thick material, which makes grinding easy. It was utilized for preparing medicine. The mortar was collected in the museum in 1957.
Preserved in Chinese Medical Association/ Museum of Chinese Medicine, Shanghai University of Traditional Chinese Medicine

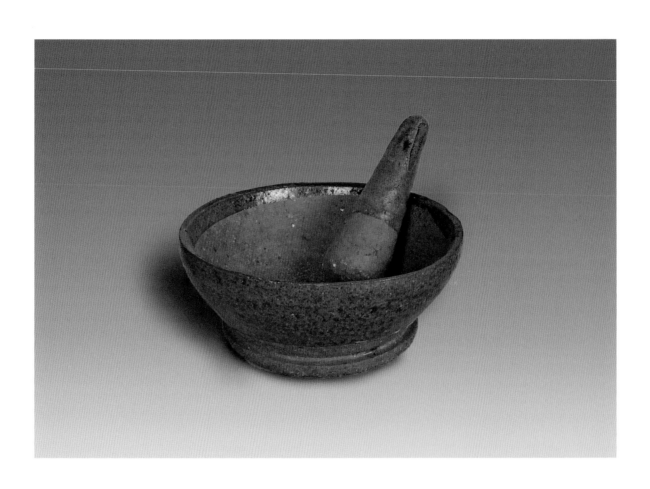

研钵

清

瓷质

口径 18.7 厘米，通高 7.6 厘米

Mortar

Qing Dynasty

Porcelain

Mouth Diameter 18.7 cm/ Height 7.6 cm

敞口，平底，圈足，带杵。由粗瓷制成，口
沿内侧及钵外上半部施黄绿釉，足及底无釉；
杵柄上半部亦施釉，工艺粗糙，但质料重实
便于研磨。为制药工具。1955 年入藏。

中华医学会 / 上海中医药大学医史博物馆藏

The rough porcelain mortar has a flared mouth,
a flat bottom and a ring foot. A pestle goes
with it. The rim's inside and the upper part of
the mortar are coated with yellowish green
glaze while its foot and bottom are exposed.
The upper part of the pestle handle is also
glazed. In spite of unrefined workmanship,
the heavy and thick material of the mortar
makes grinding easy. The mortar was utilized
for preparing medicine. It was collected in the
museum in 1955.

Preserved in Chinese Medical Association/
Museum of Chinese Medicine, Shanghai
University of Traditional Chinese Medicine

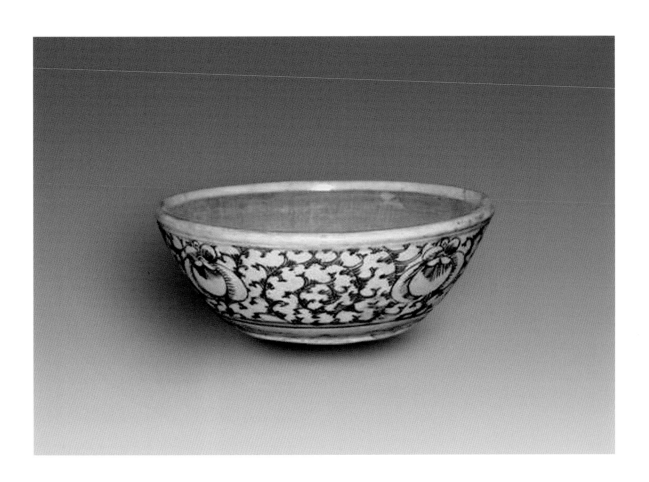

青花瓷研钵

清

瓷质

口径 26 厘米，底径 14 厘米，通高 9.5 厘米，重 1300 克

Blue-and-white Porcelain Mortar

Qing Dynasty

Porcelain

Mouth Diameter 26 cm/ Bottom Diameter 14 cm/ Height 9.5 cm/ Weight 1,300 g

侈口，斜腹，平底。器表绘青花缠枝纹。研
药药具。

陕西医史博物馆藏

The mortar has a flared mouth, an inclined belly,
and a flat bottom. Its surface is decorated with
blue-and-white intertwining branch patterns. The
mortar was utilized for porphyrizing medicinal
ingredients.

Preserved in Shaanxi Museum of Medical History

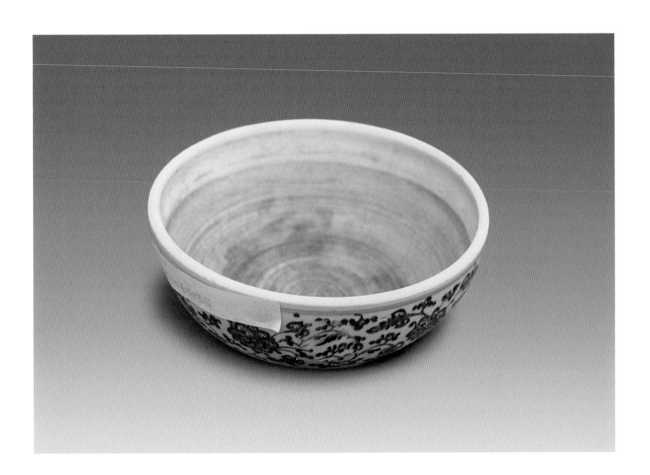

大型青花研药擂钵

清

瓷质

口外径 29.1 厘米，底径 14.3 厘米，通高 11.6 厘米，腹深 10 厘米，重 2100 克

Large Blue-and-white Mortar

Qing Dynasty

Porcelain

Mouth Outer Diameter 29.1 cm/ Bottom Diameter 14.3 cm/ Height 11.6 cm/ Belly Depth 10 cm/ Weight 2,100 g

敞口，斜腹，平底，无杵。器表绘青花花卉
图案。用于加工炮制药物。

广东中医药博物馆藏

The mortar has a flared mouth, an inclined belly and a flat bottom. There is no pestle that goes with it. Its surface is painted with blue-and-white flower patterns. The mortar was utilized for processing and preparing medicinal ingredients.

Preserved in Guangdong Chinese Medicine Museum

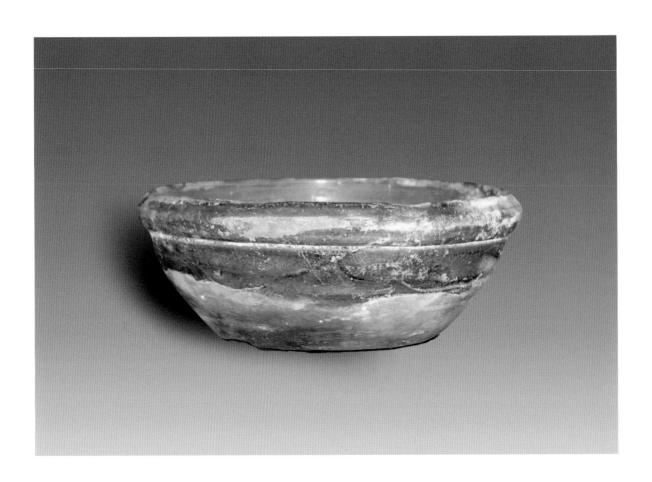

绿釉研钵

清

瓷质

口径 16 厘米，底径 10 厘米，通高 7 厘米，重 400 克

Green-glazed Mortar and Pestle

Qing Dynasty

Porcelain

Mouth Diameter 16 cm/ Bottom Diameter 10 cm/ Height 7 cm/ Weight 400 g

束口，斜腹。钵内及上腹为绿釉，下腹无釉。
研药工具。

　　　　　　陕西医史博物馆藏

The mortar has a contracted mouth and an
inclined belly. The interior and upper part of
the mortar are covered with green glaze. The
collection was used for grinding medicinal
ingredients.

Preserved in Shaanxi Museum of Medical History

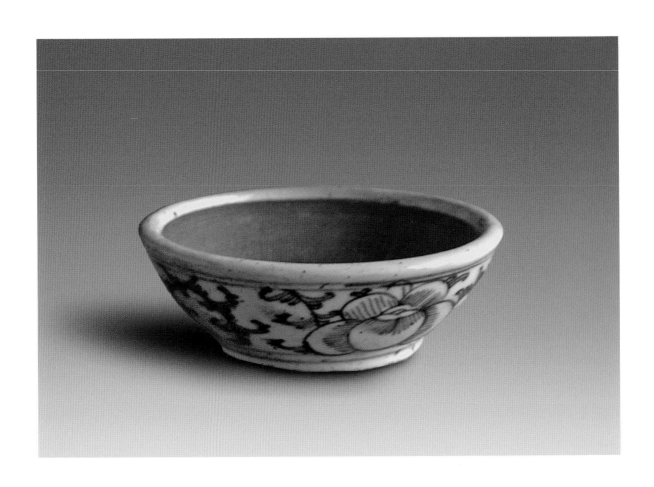

药臼

清

瓷质

口径 14 厘米，高 5 厘米

Medicine Mortar

Qing Dynasty

Porcelain

Mouth Diameter 14 cm/ Height 5 cm

敞口，腹内收，平底。外壁有青花缠枝纹饰。
研药器具。民间征集。

　　成都中医药大学中医药传统文化博物馆藏

The mortar has a flared mouth, a contracted belly, and a flat bottom. The wall is decorated with blue-and-white intertwining branch patterns. The mortar was utilized for porphyrizing medicinal ingredients. It was collected from a private owner. Preserved in Museum of Traditional Chinese Medicine Culture, Chengdu University of Traditional Chinese Medicine

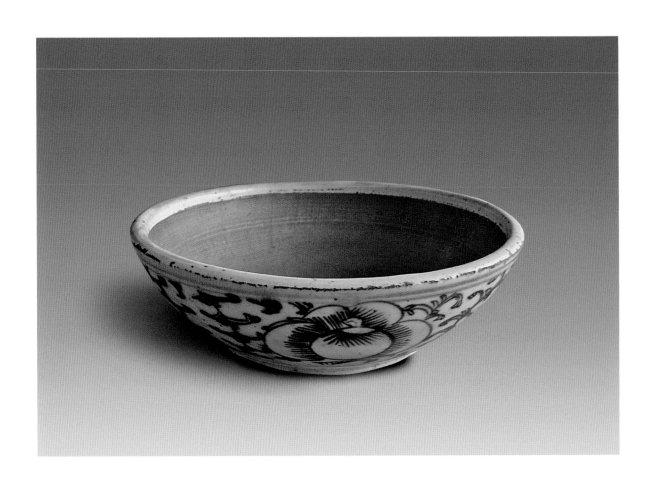

药臼

清

瓷质

口径 21 厘米，高 7 厘米

Medicine Mortar

Qing Dynasty

Porcelain

Mouth Diameter 21 cm/ Height 7 cm

敞口，斜腹，平底。外壁有青花缠枝纹饰。

研药器具。民间征集。

　成都中医药大学中医药传统文化博物馆藏

The mortar has a flared mouth, a inclined belly, and a flat bottom. Its wall is decorated with blue-and-white intertwining branch patterns. The mortar was utilized for porphyrizing medicinal ingredients. It was collected from a private owner. Preserved in Museum of Traditional Chinese Medicine Culture, Chengdu University of Traditional Chinese Medicine

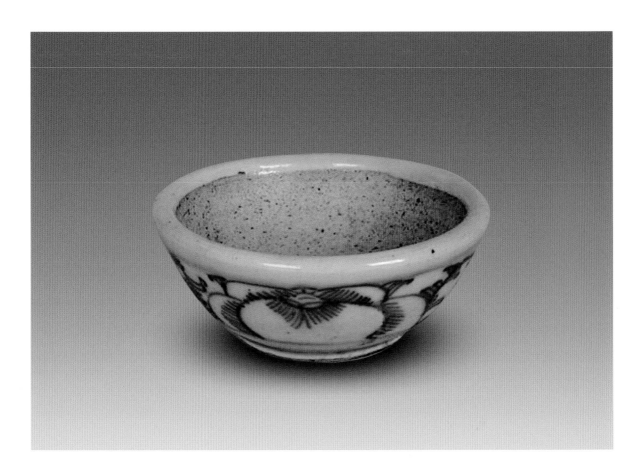

研钵

清

瓷质

口外径 10.95 厘米，底径 5.8 厘米，高 4 厘米

Mortar

Qing Dynasty

Porcelain

Mouth Outer Diameter 10.95 cm/ Bottom Diameter 5.8 cm/ Height 4 cm

敞口，平底，器表绘青花缠枝纹，底无釉无款。
制药用具。

中华医学会 / 上海中医药大学医史博物馆藏

The mortar has a flared mouth and a flat
bottom. Its surface is painted with blue-and-
white intertwining branch designs. No glaze or
inscription is on the bottom. The mortar was
utilized for preparing medicine.
Preserved in Chinese Medical Association/Museum
of Chinese Medicine, Shanghai University of
Traditional Chinese Medicine

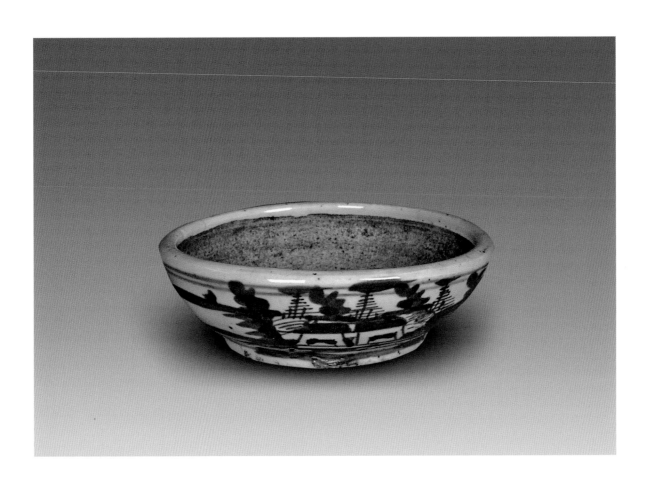

研钵

清

瓷质

口外径 13.7 厘米，底径 8.6 厘米，高 4.6 厘米

Mortar

Qing Dynasty

Porcelain

Mouth Outer Diameter 13.7 cm/ Bottom Diameter 8.6 cm/ Height 4.6 cm

敞口，平底，圈足。器表绘青花乡村风光图，
底无釉无款，工艺粗糙。制药工具。

中华医学会 / 上海中医药大学医史博物馆藏

The porcelain mortar has a flared mouth, a flat
bottom, and a ring foot. Its surface is decorated
with blue-and-white country landscape, but
there is no glaze or inscription on the bottom.
Its workmanship is rough. The mortar was
utilized for preparing medicine.
Preserved in Chinese Medical Association/ Museum
of Chinese Medicine, Shanghai University of
Traditional Chinese Medicine

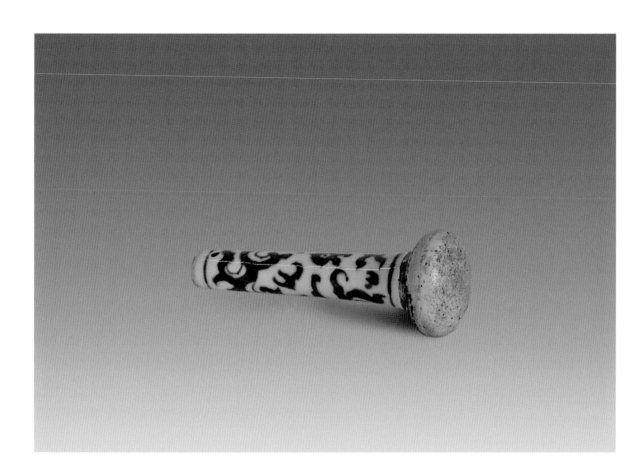

青瓷研杵

清

瓷质

通长 11.2 厘米，头径 3.7 厘米，柄径 1.6 厘米

Celadon Pestle

Qing Dynasty

Porcelain

Length 11.2 cm/ Head Diameter 3.7 cm/ Handle Diameter 1.6 cm

表面绘青花云龙图案。制药工具。

中华医学会 / 上海中医药大学医史博物馆藏

The surface of the pestle is painted with blue-and-white dragon among clouds designs. The pestle was utilized for preparing medicine.
Preserved in Chinese Medical Association/ Museum of Chinese Medicine, Shanghai University of Traditional Chinese Medicine

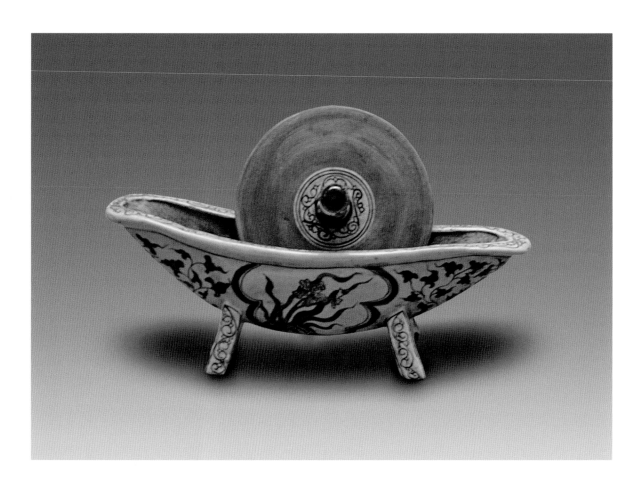

药碾

清

瓷质

长 32 厘米，宽 7 厘米，高 9.5 厘米

Medicine Groove

Qing Dynasty

Porcelain

Length 32 cm/ Width 7 cm/ Height 9.5 cm

平口，半圆形腹，饰青花纹饰。保存完好。
由民间征集。

　　成都中医药大学中医药传统文化博物馆藏

The groove has a flat mouth and a semiannular
belly with blue-and-white flower patterns.
It was collected from a private owner and is
basically in good condition.
Preserved in Museum of Traditional Chinese
Medicine Culture, Chengdu University of
Traditional Chinese Medicine

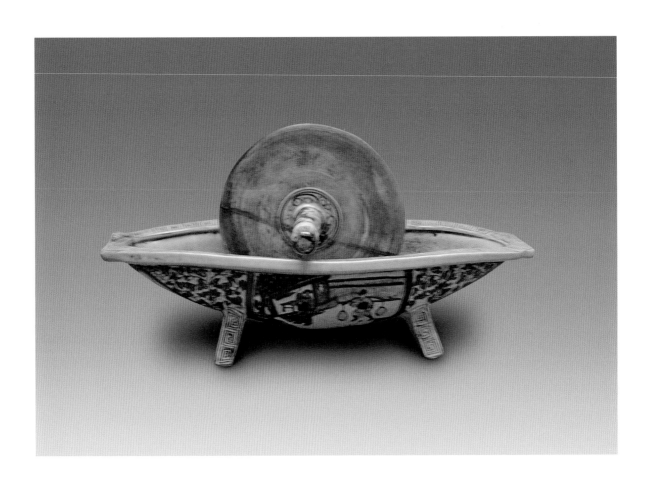

药碾

清

瓷质

长 36 厘米，宽 8.5 厘米，高 11 厘米，轮径 17 厘米

Medicine Groove

Qing Dynasty

Porcelain

Length 36 cm/ Width 8.5 cm/ Height 11 cm/ Wheel Diameter 17 cm

呈船形，平口，半圆形腹，八字形对足。口部饰青花回形纹，腹部饰青花人物和缠枝花纹，足部亦绘有青花缠枝纹和回形纹，碾轮中上部位及把手饰有青花缠枝纹。用于碾磨药物，是常见的中药加工用具。造型精美，保存完好。由民间征集。

成都中医药大学中医药传统文化博物馆藏

The groove is shaped like a boat with a flat mouth, a semiannular belly and splayed feet. Its rim is adorned with blue-and-white fret patterns. Its belly is adorned with blue-and-white figures and intertwining branches. Its feet are also decorated with blue-and-white intertwining branches and fret patterns while its handles and the upper and middle parts of its wheels are decorated with blue-and-white intertwining branch patterns. The groove was a common tool for processing traditional Chinese medicine. It was collected from a private owner and is still in good condition with exquisite styling.

Preserved in Museum of Traditional Chinese Medicine Culture, Chengdu University of Traditional Chinese Medicine

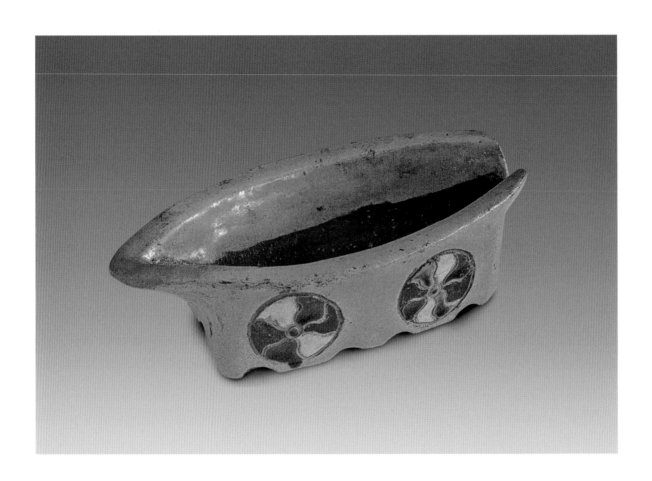

石湾窑三彩药碾

清

瓷质

长 23 厘米，宽 13 厘米，高 6 厘米

Tri-colored Medicine Groove of Shiwan Kiln

Qing Dynasty

Porcelain

Length 23 cm/ Width 13 cm/ Height 6 cm

口呈小船形，上宽下窄成槽形，长方形座。胎体厚重，造型古朴，施粉蓝色釉，两边各饰蓝、白、绿三彩相间的团花二朵。为广东石湾窑制的碾药用器，该形制传世器甚少。

邓禹藏

The medicine groove has a boat-shaped mouth. Its swelling body, which tapers downwards, resembles a slot with a rectangular base. The groove is thickly potted in simple style and coated with pale blue glaze. It is decorated with patterns of two tri-colored flowers in blue, white and green on both sides. The groove, which was made in Shiwan Kiln in Guangdong Province, was utilized for crushing medicine. Very few grooves of this type have been handed down.

Collected by Deng Yu

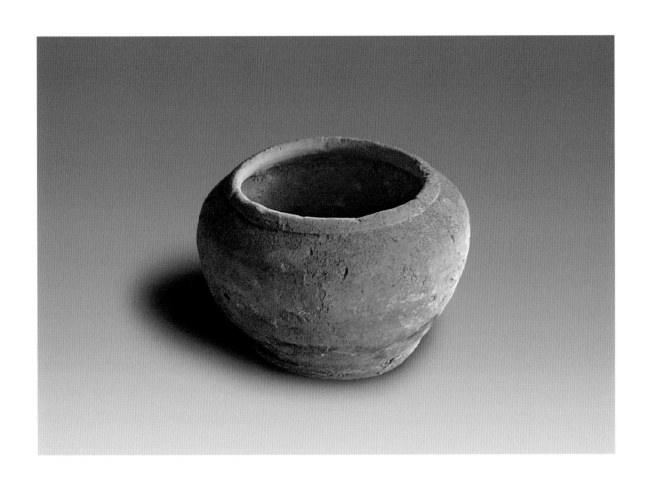

药坛

清

陶质

口径 11 厘米，底径 10 厘米，高 11 厘米

Medicine Pot

Qing Dynasty

Pottery

Mouth Diameter 11 cm/ Bottom Diameter 10 cm/ Height 11 cm

敛口，鼓腹，平底。由民间征集。

成都中医药大学中医药传统文化博物馆藏

The medicine pot has a contracted mouth, a bulged belly, and a flat bottom. It was collected from a private owner.

Preserved in Museum of Traditional Chinese Medicine Culture, Chengdu University of Traditional Chinese Medicine

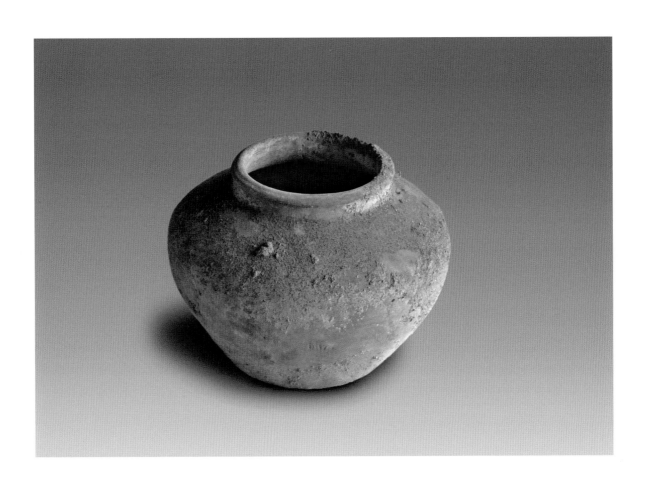

药坛

清

陶质

口径 10 厘米，底径 11 厘米，高 14 厘米

Medicine Pot

Qing Dynasty

Pottery

Mouth Diameter 10 cm/ Bottom Diameter 11 cm/ Height 14 cm

直口，鼓肩，腹内收，平底。由民间征集。

成都中医药大学中医药传统文化博物馆藏

The medicine pot has a vertical mouth, a bulged shoulder, a contracted belly, and a flat bottom. It was collected from a private owner.

Preserved in Museum of Traditional Chinese Medicine Culture, Chengdu University of Traditional Chinese Medicine

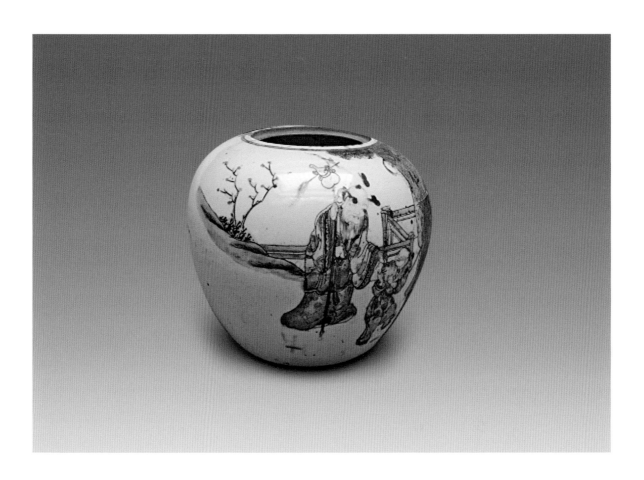

药坛

清

瓷质

口径 9.5 厘米，腹径 23 厘米，高 19 厘米

Medicine Jar

Qing Dynasty

Porcelain

Mouth Diameter 9.5 cm/ Belly Diameter 23 cm/ Height 19 cm

敛口，鼓腹，平底。饰五彩人物图案。保存
完整，由民间征集。

　成都中医药大学中医药传统文化博物馆藏

The medicine jar has a contracted mouth, a
bulged belly, and a flat bottom. It is painted
with patterns of multi-colored figures. It was
collected from a private owner and is still in
good condition.

Preserved in Museum of Traditional Chinese
Medicine Culture, Chengdu University of
Traditional Chinese Medicine

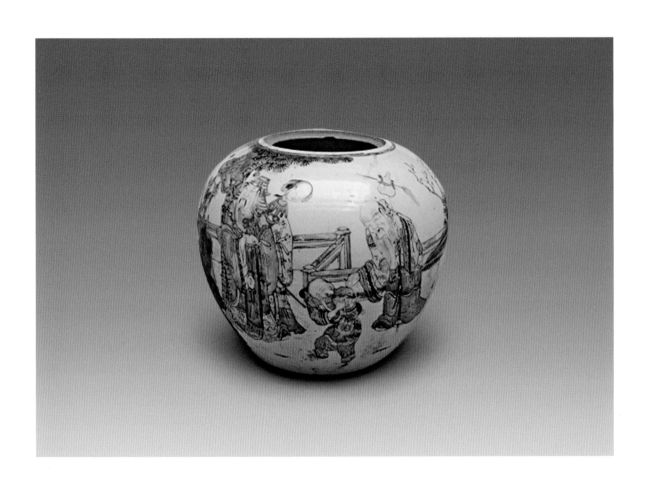

药坛

清

瓷质

口径 9.5 厘米，腹径 23 厘米，高 19 厘米

Medicine Jar

Qing Dynasty

Porcelain

Mouth Diameter 9.5 cm/ Belly Diameter 23 cm/ Height 19 cm

敛口，鼓腹，平底。饰五彩人物图案。保存完整，由民间征集。

成都中医药大学中医药传统文化博物馆藏

The medicine jar has a contracted mouth, a bulged belly, and a flat bottom. It is painted with patterns of multi-colored figures. It was collected from a private owner and is still in good condition.

Preserved in Museum of Traditional Chinese Medicine Culture, Chengdu University of Traditional Chinese Medicine

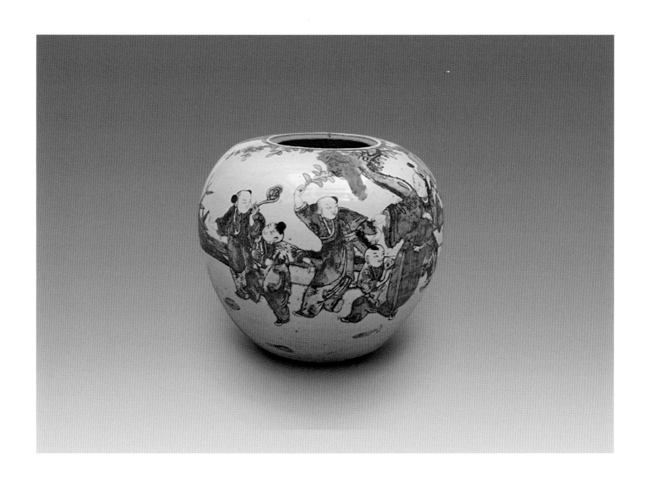

药坛

清

瓷质

口径 9.5 厘米，腹径 23 厘米，高 19 厘米

Medicine Jar

Qing Dynasty

Porcelain

Diameter 9.5 cm/ Belly Diameter 23 cm/ Height 19 cm

敛口，鼓腹，平底。饰五彩人物图案。保存
完整。由民间征集。

成都中医药大学中医药传统文化博物馆藏

The medicine jar has a contracted mouth, a
bulged belly, and a flat bottom. It is painted
with patterns of multi-colored figures. It was
collected from a private owner and is still in
good condition.

Preserved in Museum of Traditional Chinese
Medicine Culture, Chengdu University of
Traditional Chinese Medicine

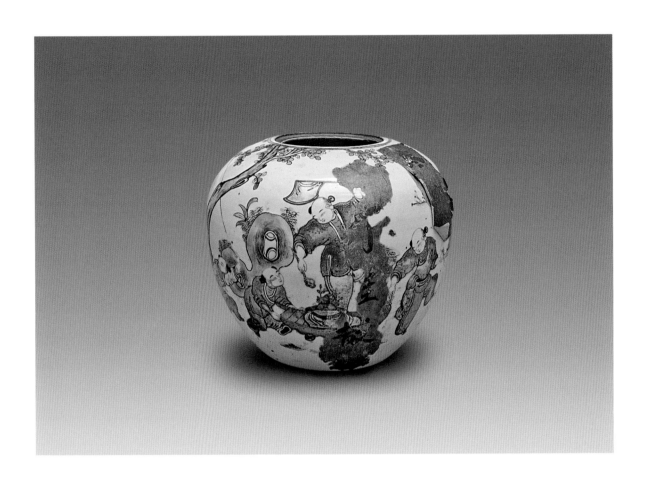

药坛

清

瓷质

口径 9.5 厘米，腹径 23 厘米，高 19 厘米

Medicine Jar

Qing Dynasty

Porcelain

Mouth Diameter 9.5 cm/ Belly Diameter 23 cm/ Height 19 cm

敛口，鼓腹，平底。饰五彩人物图案。保存
完整，由民间征集。

成都中医药大学中医药传统文化博物馆藏

The medicine jar has a contracted mouth, a
bulged belly, and a flat bottom. It is painted
with patterns of multi-colored figures. It was
collected from a private owner and is still in
good condition.

Preserved in Museum of Traditional Chinese
Medicine Culture, Chengdu University of
Traditional Chinese Medicine

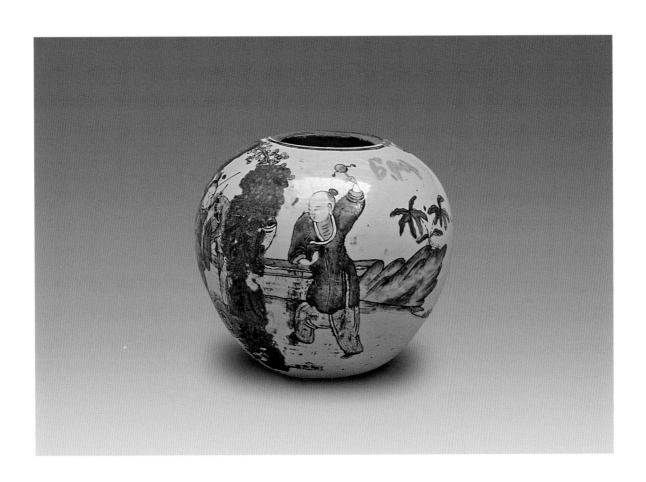

药坛

清

瓷质

口径 9.5 厘米，腹径 23 厘米，高 19 厘米

Medicine Jar

Qing Dynasty

Porcelain

Mouth Diameter 9.5 cm/ Belly Diameter 23 cm/ Height 19 cm

敛口，鼓腹，平底，盖已失。红胎白釉，绘五彩人物图案，人物活泼生动，色泽鲜艳而层次分明。坛上有纸贴标签，书有"调气散""苏菀"等字，应为盛装药物用品，此形制在川西中药房中十分常见。民间征集。

成都中医药大学中医药传统文化博物馆藏

The jar has a contracted mouth, a bulged belly and a flat bottom. And the lid is missing. It is covered with white glaze and is painted with patterns of colorful and lively figures. The picture has bright colors and distinct layers. There is a paper label with characters reading "Tiao Qi San" (qi-regulating powder) and "Su Wan" etc. The jar was used for containing medicine. Jars of this shape were very common in Chinese medicine drug stores in the western region of Sichuan Province. The jar was collected from a private owner.

Preserved in Museum of Traditional Chinese Medicine Culture, Chengdu University of Traditional Chinese Medicine

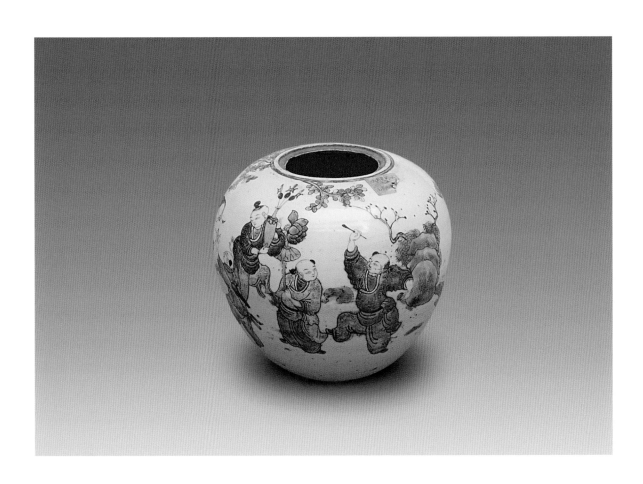

药坛

清

瓷质

口径 9.5 厘米，腹径 23 厘米，高 19 厘米

Medicine Jar

Qing Dynasty

Porcelain

Mouth Diameter 9.5 cm/ Belly Diameter 23 cm/ Height 19 cm

敛口，鼓腹，平底。饰五彩人物图案。保存
完整。由民间征集。

　　成都中医药大学中医药传统文化博物馆藏

The jar has a contracted mouth, a bulged
belly, and a flat bottom. It is painted with
patterns of five-colored character figures. The
jar was collected from a private owner and is
still in good condition.

Preserved in Museum of Traditional Chinese
Medicine Culture, Chengdu University of
Traditional Chinese Medicine

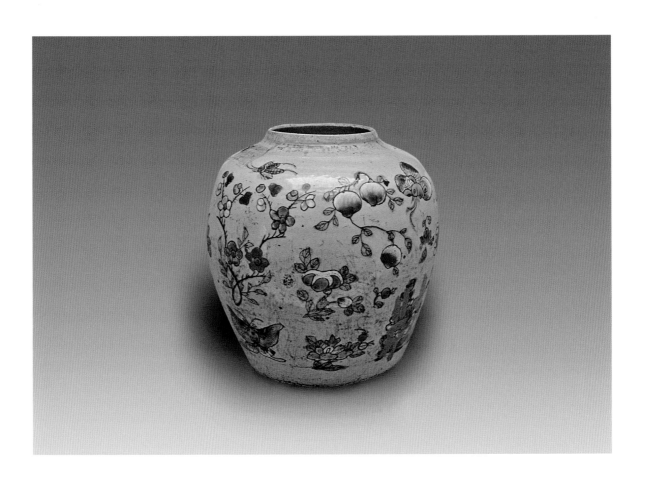

药坛

清

瓷质

口径 9.5 厘米，底径 17 厘米，高 16 厘米

Medicine Jar

Qing Dynasty

Porcelain

Mouth Diameter 9.5 cm/ Bottom Diameter 17 cm/ Height 16 cm

直口，鼓肩，直腹，平底。施黄釉，饰粉彩桃叶纹饰，图案简洁，色彩艳丽而明快，器形端庄。保存较好。由民间征集。

成都中医药大学中医药传统文化博物馆藏

The jar has a vertical mouth, a bulged shoulder, a straight belly, and a flat bottom. It is coated with yellow glaze and decorated with powder-enameled peach leaf patterns. The picture is colorful and bright, and the shape of the jar is dignified. The jar was collected from a private owner and is still in good condition.

Preserved in Museum of Traditional Chinese Medicine Culture, Chengdu University of Traditional Chinese Medicine

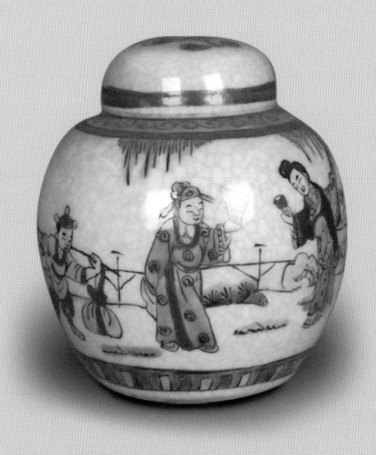

瓷药坛

清

瓷质

口内径 3.6 厘米，口外径 4.4 厘米，腹径 10.4 厘米，高 11.4 厘米

坛形，直口，圈足，平底，上配扣盖。通身开片，坛表面彩绘人物故事画，底无款识，工艺精细。盛药器具。

中华医学会／上海中医药大学医史博物馆藏

Porcelain Medicine Jar

Qing Dynasty

Porcelain

Mouth Inner Diameter 3.6 cm/ Mouth Outer Diameter 4.4 cm/ Belly Diameter 10.4 cm/ Height 11.4 cm

The jar has a lid, a vertical mouth, a flat bottom, and a ring foot. The surface of the jar is painted with story pictures. There is no inscription on the bottom. The pot was used for containing medicine.

Preserved in Chinese Medical Association/ Museum of Chinese Medicine, Shanghai University of Traditional Chinese Medicine

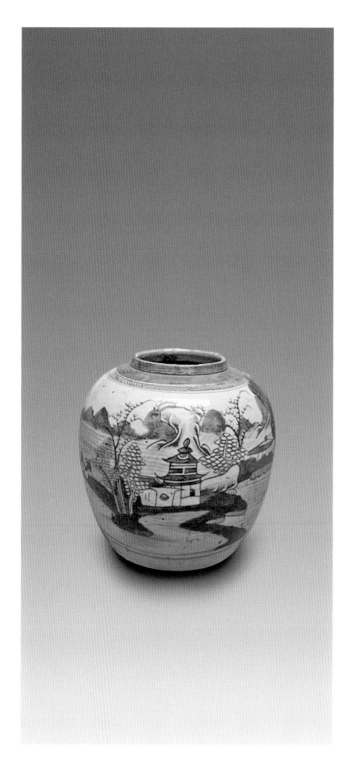

药坛

清

瓷质

口径 19 厘米，底径 17.5 厘米，高 21 厘米

直口，鼓腹，平底。饰青花山水纹饰。保存
完好。由民间征集。

　　成都中医药大学中医药传统文化博物馆藏

Medicine Jar

Qing Dynasty

Porcelain

Mouth Diameter 19 cm/ Bottom Diameter 17.5 cm/
Height 21 cm

The jar has a vertical mouth, a bulged belly,
and a flat bottom. It is painted with blue-and-
white landscape. It was collected from a private
owner and is still in good condition.

Preserved in Museum of Traditional Chinese
Medicine Culture, Chengdu University of
Traditional Chinese Medicine

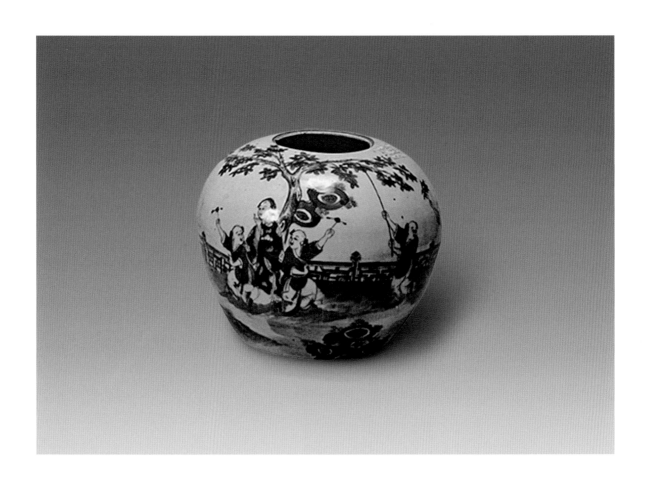

青花人物药坛

清

瓷质

腹径 26 厘米，高 21 厘米

Medicine Jar with Blue-and-white Figures

Qing Dynasty

Porcelain

Belly Diameter 26 cm/ Height 21 cm

敛口，圆唇，丰肩，平底。白底青花，图案
佳美。以盛放易潮湿的种子类药为主。

　　成都中医药大学中医药传统文化博物馆藏

The jar has a contracted mouth, a round rim, a
plump shoulder, a flat bottom and a ring foot.
Its white background is painted with beautiful
blue patterns. It was used for storing seed drugs
which get moisturized easily.
Preserved in Museum of Traditional Chinese
Medicine Culture, Chengdu University of
Traditional Chinese Medicine

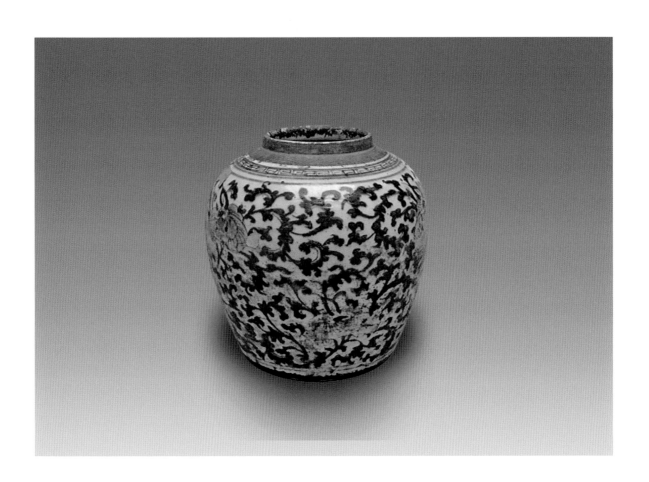

药坛

清

瓷质

口径 9 厘米，底径 17 厘米，高 20 厘米

Medicine Jar

Qing Dynasty

Porcelain

Mouth Diameter 9 cm/ Bottom Diameter 17 cm/ Height 20 cm

直口，鼓腹，平底。饰青花枝叶纹，釉色莹润，纹饰色彩艳丽。保存完好。由民间征集。

成都中医药大学中医药传统文化博物馆藏

The jar has a vertical mouth, a bulged belly, and a flat bottom. It is decorated with brilliant blue-and-white foliage patterns. The glaze is mellow and shiny. The jar was collected from a private owner and is still in good condition.

Preserved in Museum of Traditional Chinese Medicine Culture, Chengdu University of Traditional Chinese Medicine

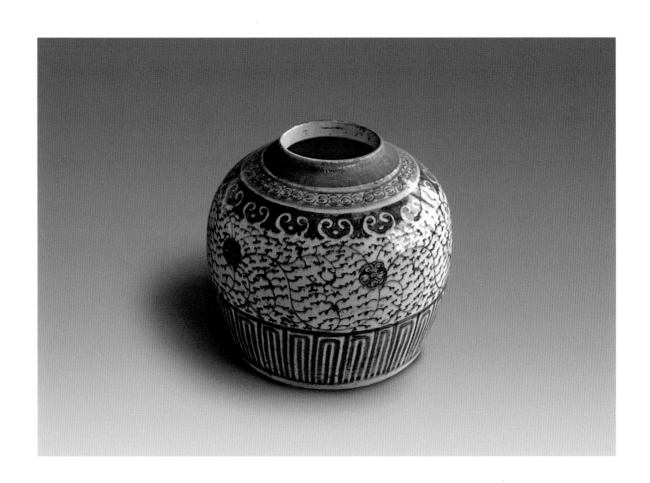

药坛

清

瓷质

口径 9 厘米，底径 17 厘米，高 20 厘米

Medicine Jar

Qing Dynasty

Porcelain

Mouth Diameter 9 cm/ Bottom Diameter 17 cm/ Height 20 cm

鼓肩，直腹，圈足。饰青花缠枝纹和回纹。
由民间征集。

　　成都中医药大学中医药传统文化博物馆藏

The jar has a bulged shoulder, a vertical belly
and a ring foot. It is decorated with blue-and-
white intertwining branch patterns and fret
patterns. The jar was collected from a private
owner.

Preserved in Museum of Traditional Chinese
Medicine Culture, Chengdu University of
Traditional Chinese Medicine

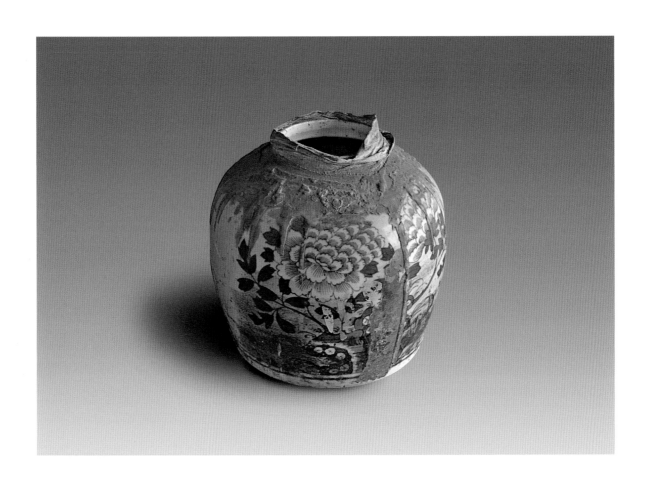

药坛

清

瓷质

口径 10 厘米，底径 11 厘米，高 14 厘米

Medicine Jar

Qing Dynasty

Porcelain

Mouth Diameter 10 cm/ Bottom Diameter 11 cm/ Height 14 cm

直口，鼓肩，腹内收，平底。饰青花花卉纹。
由民间征集。

　　成都中医药大学中医药传统文化博物馆藏

The jar has a vertical mouth, a bulged shoulder,
a downwand-contracted belly, and a flat bottom.
It is decorated with blue-and-white floral patterns.
The jar was collected from a private owner.
Preserved in Museum of Traditional Chinese
Medicine Culture, Chengdu University of
Traditional Chinese Medicine

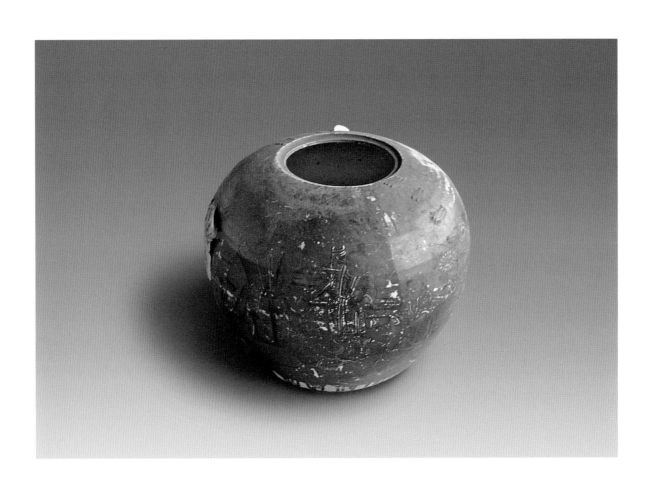

药坛

清

瓷质

口径 10 厘米，底径 14 厘米，高 19 厘米

Medicine Jar

Qing Dynasty

Porcelain

Mouth Diameter 10 cm/ Bottom Diameter 14 cm/ Height 19 cm

鼓腹，平底，盖已失。饰青花人物图案，被
人为漆上一层红漆。由民间征集。

成都中医药大学中医药传统文化博物馆藏

The jar has a bulged belly and a flat bottom.
The lid is missing. It is decorated with blue-
and-white patterned figures and later painted
red on the upper layer. The jar was collected
from a private owner.

Preserved in Museum of Traditional Chinese
Medicine Culture, Chengdu University of
Traditional Chinese Medicine

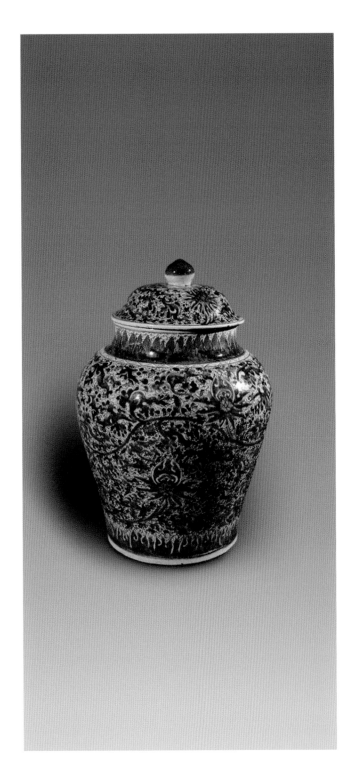

青花加彩大药坛

清

瓷质

口径 23 厘米，底径 27 厘米，高 57 厘米

Big Blue-and-white Medicine Jar

Qing Dynasty

Porcelain

Mouth Diameter 23 cm/ Bottom Diameter 27 cm/

Height 57 cm

直口，高领，鼓肩，平底，带盖，盖顶宝珠纽。

通体饰青花釉里红缠枝花卉纹，造型华丽。

中华医学会 / 上海中医药大学医史博物馆藏

The jar has a vertical mouth, a long neck, a
bulged shoulder, and a flat bottom. The top
of its lid has a pearl-shaped knob. The jar is
coated with blue-and-white glaze and decorated
with red intertwining floral patterns. It has a
gorgeous styling.

Preserved in Chinese Medical Association/ Museum
of Chinese Medicine, Shanghai University of
Traditional Chinese Medicine

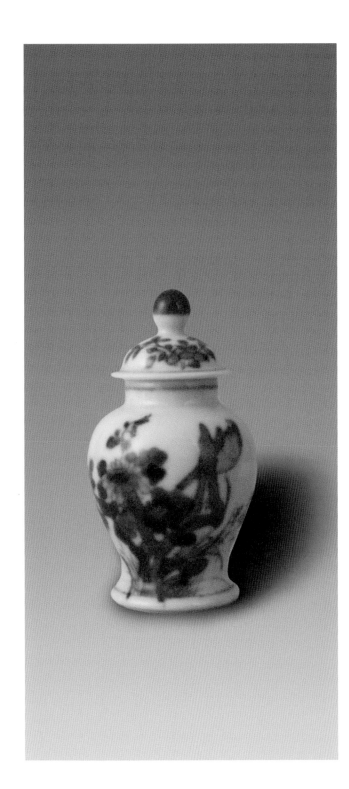

药坛

清

瓷质

腹径 5.9 厘米，底径 4 厘米，通高 9.7 厘米

Medicine Jar

Qing Dynasty

Porcelain

Belly Diameter 5.9 cm/ Bottom Diameter 4 cm/

Height 9.7 cm

坛形，直口，高领，鼓肩，平底，带盖，盖顶球形纽。器表绘青花菊兰立鸟图案，工艺佳，造型美观。盛药器具。

中华医学会／上海中医药大学医史博物馆藏

The jar has a vertical mouth, a long neck, a bulged shoulder and a flat bottom. The top of its lid is a spherical knob. The jar is painted with blue-and-white chrysanthemum and bird patterns. The jar has exquisite craftsmanship and beautiful styling. It was used for containing medicine.

Preserved in Chinese Medical Association/ Museum of Chinese Medicine, Shanghai University of Traditional Chinese Medicine

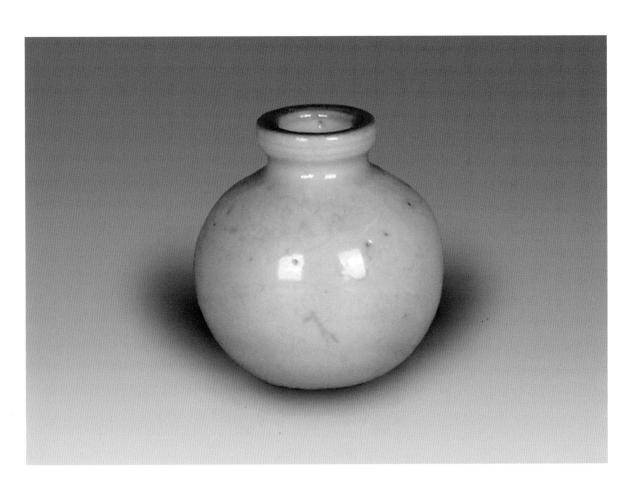

瓷药坛

清

瓷质

口内径 1.55 厘米，口外径 2.6 厘米，腹径 5.35 厘米，高 5.4 厘米

Porcelain Medicine Jar

Qing Dynasty

Porcelain

Mouth Inner Diameter 1.55 cm/ Mouth Outer Diameter 2.6 cm/ Belly Diameter 5.35 cm/ Height 5.4 cm

坛形，直口，鼓腹，平底，通身施青灰釉，釉下浅刻各式花纹，口沿涂浅黄色釉，底无釉无款，工艺较好。盛药用具。

中华医学会 / 上海中医药大学医史博物馆藏

The jar has a vertical mouth, a bulged belly and a flat bottom. The body is coated with gray glaze while the rim is covered with light yellow glaze. Underneath the glaze are various flower patterns. There is no glaze or seal mark on the bottom. The exquisite jar was used for containing medicine.

Preserved in Chinese Medical Association/ Museum of Chinese Medicine, Shanghai University of Traditional Chinese Medicine

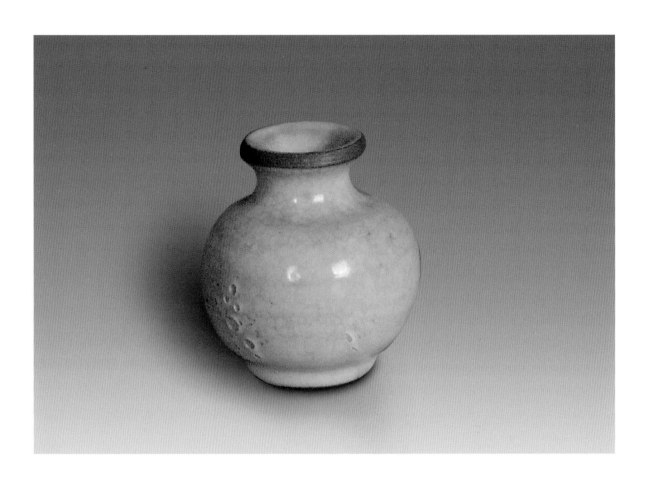

药坛

清

瓷质

口内径 1.35 厘米，口外径 3.5 厘米，腹径 6.15 厘米

Medicine Jar

Qing Dynasty

Porcelain

Mouth Inner Diameter 1.35 cm/ Mouth Outer Diameter 3.5 cm/ Belly Diameter 6.15 cm

坛形，平底，圈足。通体施灰白色釉，但底部无釉，也无题记。盛药器具。

中华医学会 / 上海中医药大学医史博物馆藏

The jar has a flat base and a ring foot. Its body is coated with grayish white glaze but there is no glaze or inscription on the bottom. The jar was used for storing medicine.

Preserved in Chinese Medical Association/ Museum of Chinese Medicine, Shanghai University of Traditional Chinese Medicine

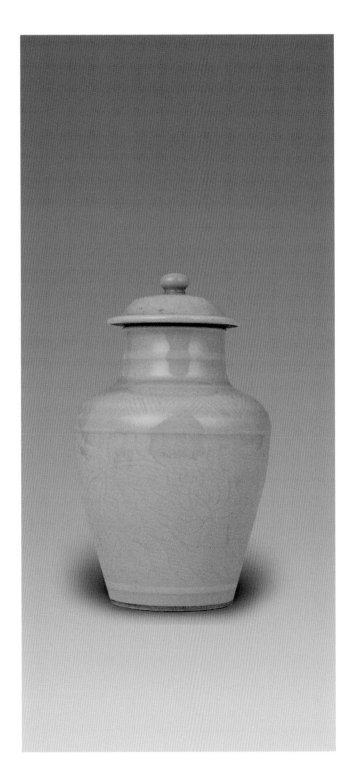

药坛

清

瓷质

口径4.6厘米，腹径8.8厘米，底径5.4厘米，

通高14.6厘米

Medicine Jar

Qing Dynasty

Porcelain

Mouth Diameter 4.6 cm/ Belly Diameter 8.8 cm/

Bottom Diameter 5.4 cm/ Height 14.6 cm

圆瓶形，直口，平底，配扣盖，盖上置圆纽。
通体青绿釉，工艺精细，美观大方。盛药器具。

中华医学会／上海中医药大学医史博物馆藏

The round jar has a vertical mouth and a flat
bottom. The top of its lid is a hemispherical
knob. The jar is coated with green glaze.
The exquisite and elegant jar was used for
containing medicine.
Preserved in Chinese Medical Association/ Museum
of Chinese Medicine, Shanghai University of
Traditional Chinese Medicine

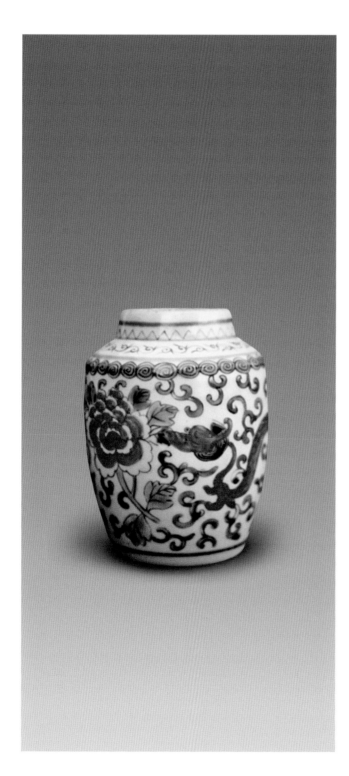

五彩药用盖罐

清

瓷质

口外径 4.6 厘米，腹径 7.8 厘米，底径 5.1 厘米，

高 9.8 厘米，腹深 9.3 厘米，重 380 克

Colorful Medicine Jar

Qing Dynasty

Porcelain

Mouth Outer Diameter 4.6 cm/ Belly Diameter

7.8 cm/ Bottom Diameter 5.1 cm/ Height 9.8 cm/

Belly Depth 9.3 cm/ Weight 380 g

直口，折肩，鼓腹，平底。器表绘五彩龙纹
和花卉图案。用于盛药物。

　　　　　　　　　　　广东中医药博物馆藏

The jar has a vertical mouth, a folded shoulder,
a bulged belly and a flat bottom. Its surface is
painted with multi-colored dragon and flower
patterns. The jar was used for storing medicine.
Preserved in Guangdong Chinese Medicine Museum

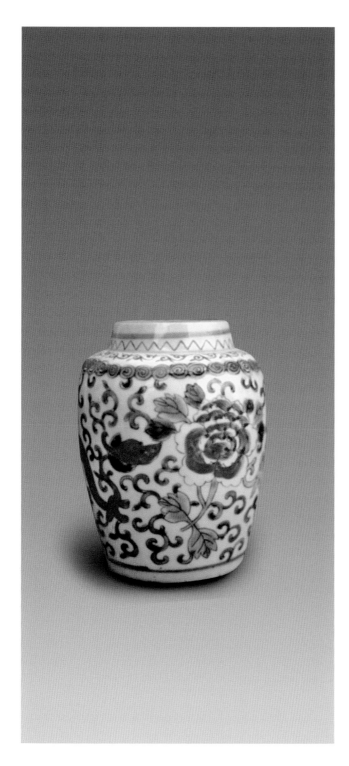

五彩药用盖罐

清

陶瓷质

口外径 4.46 厘米，腹径 7.95 厘米，底径
5.45 厘米，通高 10 厘米，腹深 8.7 厘米，
重 417.5 克

Colorful Medicine Jar

Qing Dynasty

Porcelain

Mouth Outer Diameter 4.46 cm/ Belly Diameter
7.95 cm/ Bottom Diameter 5.45 cm/ Height 10 cm/
Belly Depth 8.7 cm/ Weight 417.5 g

直口，折肩，鼓腹，平底。器表绘五彩龙纹
和花卉图案。用于盛药物。

广东中医药博物馆藏

The jar has a vertical mouth, a folded shoulder,
a bulged belly and a flat bottom. Its surface is
painted with multi-colored dragon and flower
patterns. The jar was used for storing medicine.
Preserved in Guangdong Chinese Medicine Museum

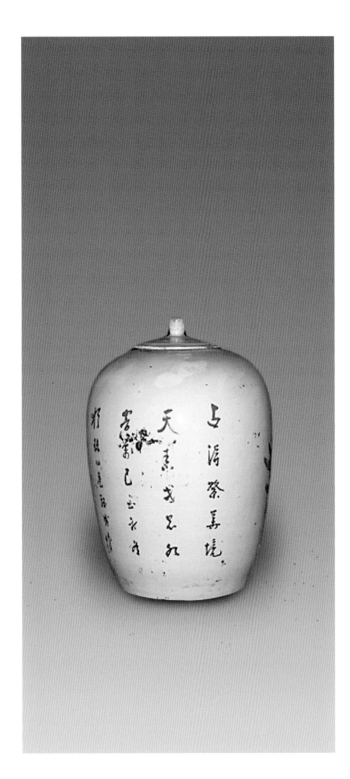

彩花药罐

清

瓷质

口径 9.5 厘米，底径 15.5 厘米，通高 28.5

厘米，重 2600 克

Colorful Medicine Pot

Qing Dynasty

Porcelain

Mouth Diameter 9.5 cm/ Bottom Diameter 15.5 cm/

Height 28.5 cm/ Weight 2,600 g

子母口，直腹，圈足。通体豆青色底，器壁
有牡丹喜鹊图题诗。贮药器物。

陕西医史博物馆藏

The pot has a snap-lid, a vertical belly and a
ring foot. Its whole body is bean green. Its wall
is decorated with peony and magpie designs
accompanied with a related poem. The pot was
used for storing medicine.

Preserved in Shaanxi Museum of Medical History

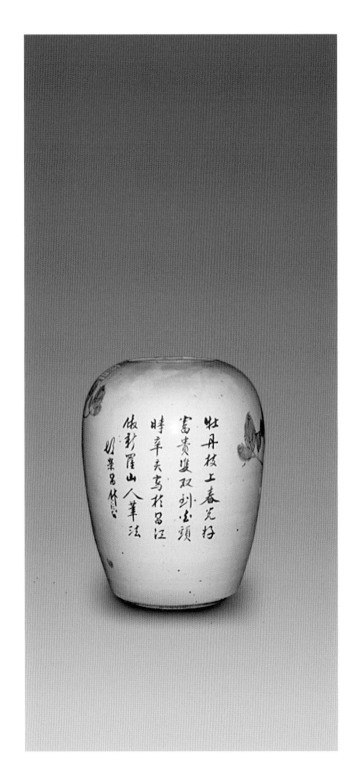

彩花药罐

清

瓷质

口径 10 厘米，底径 15 厘米，通高 28.5 厘米，

重 2500 克

Colorful Medicine Pot

Qing Dynasty

Porcelain

Mouth Diameter 10 cm/ Bottom Diameter 15 cm/

Height 28.5 cm/ Weight 2,500 g

子母口，直腹，圈足。通体豆青色底，器壁有牡丹小鸟红梅图题诗。贮药器具。陕西西安藻露堂中药店征集。

陕西医史博物馆藏

The pot has a snap-lid, a vertical belly and a ring foot. Its body is pea green. Its wall is decorated with peony, bird and red plum designs accompanied with a related poem. The pot was used for storing medicine. It was collected from Zao Lu Tang Drugstore of Chinese Medicine in Xi'an, Shaanxi Province.

Preserved in Shaanxi Museum of Medical History

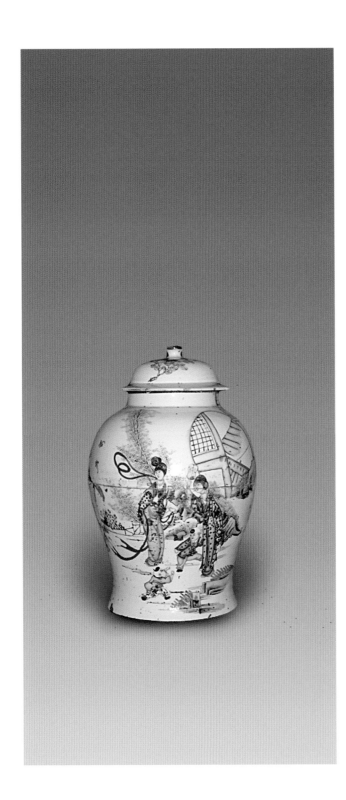

彩花大瓷瓶

清

瓷质

口径13厘米，底径20.05厘米，通高24厘米，

重 5000 克

Colorful Porcelain Bottle

Qing Dynasty

Porcelain

Mouth Diameter 13 cm/ Bottom Diameter

20.05 cm/ Height 24 cm/ Weight 5,000 g

子母口，圆肩，圆腹，圈足，带盖，腹有修补。通体豆绿色底，器壁绘两仕女戏蝶图。贮药器物。陕西西安藻露堂中药店征集。

陕西医史博物馆藏

The bottle has a snap-lid, a round shoulder, a round belly, and a ring foot. There are some repairing marks on the belly. The whole body is pea green. The wall of the bottle is painted with patterns of two elegant ladies chasing butterflies. The bottle was used for storing medicine. It was collected from Zao Lu Tang Drugstore of Chinese Medicine in Xi'an, Shaanxi Province.

Preserved in Shaanxi Museum of Medical History

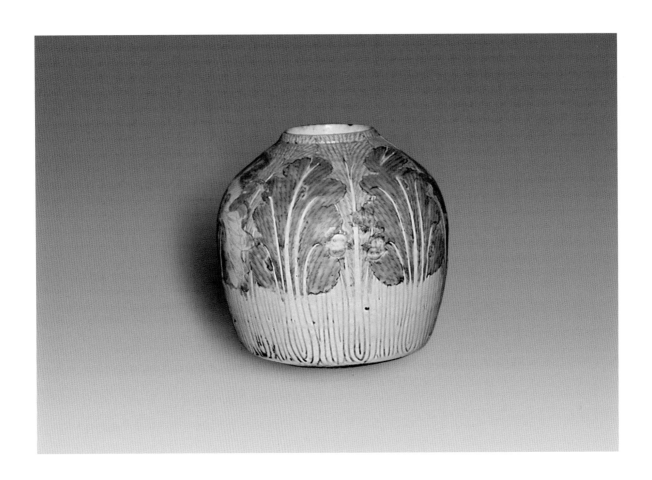

彩花药罐

清

瓷质

口径 8.5 厘米，底径 18 厘米，通高 20.5 厘米，重 2200 克

Colorful Medicine Jar

Qing Dynasty

Porcelain

Mouth Diameter 8.5 cm/ Bottom Diameter 18 cm/ Height 20.5 cm/ Weight 2,200 g

束口，圆肩，圆腹，圈足。器表彩绘绿白菜红蝴蝶图案。贮药器物。陕西西安藻露堂中药店征集。

陕西医史博物馆藏

The jar has a contracted mouth, a round shoulder, a round belly and a ring foot. Its surface is painted with green Chinese cabbages and red butterflies. The jar was used for storing medicine. It was collected from Zao Lu Tang Drugstore of Chinese Medicine in Xi'an, Shaanxi Province.

Preserved in Shaanxi Museum of Medical History

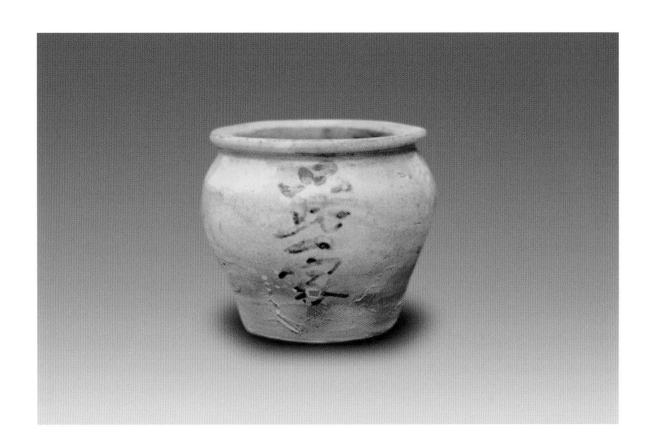

天德堂小药罐

清

瓷质

口外径 7.05 厘米，腹径 7.77 厘米，底径 5.25 厘米，通高 6.4 厘米，腹深 5.9 厘米，重 125 克

Small Medicine Jar of "Tian De Tang"

Qing Dynasty

Porcelain

Mouth Outer Diameter 7.05 cm/ Belly Diameter 7.77 cm/ Bottom Diameter 5.25 cm/ Height 6.4 cm/ Belly Depth 5.9 cm/ Weight 125 g

侈口，鼓腹，平底。器表两面书"天德堂""只
此一家"款识，为道光年间制品。用于盛药。

　　　　　　　　广东中医药博物馆藏

The jar has an wide flared mouth, a bulged belly
and a flat bottom. The two sides of the jar are
painted with characters reading "Tian De Tang"
(the name of the drug store), and "Zhi Ci Yi Jia"
(the only store) indicating that the jar was made
in Daoguang Reign of the Qing Dynasty. The jar
was used for storing medicine.

Preserved in Guangdong Chinese Medicine Museum

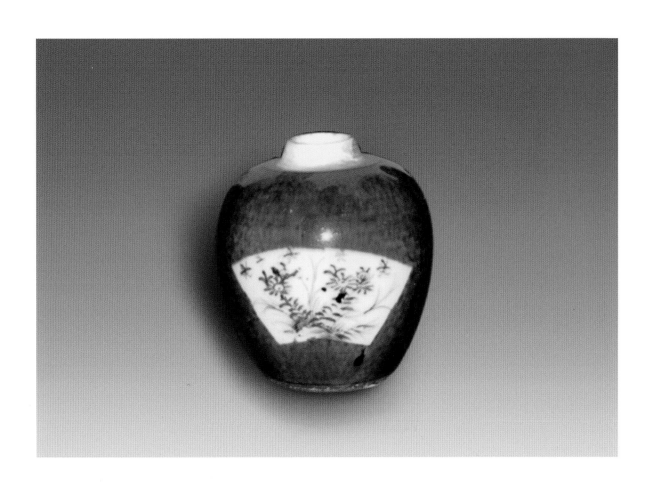

瓷药罐

清

瓷质

口径 2.8 厘米，底径 5.1 厘米，通高 9.5 厘米，重 250 克

Porcelain Medicine Jar

Qing Dynasty

Porcelain

Mouth Diameter 2.8 cm/ Bottom Diameter 5.1 cm/ Height 9.5 cm/ Weight 250 g

子母口，圆肩，圈足。通体饰蓝釉，器表两
面各绘有一扇面，其上绘兰花图。盛贮器。

陕西医史博物馆藏

The jar has a snap-lid, a round shoulder and a
ring foot. Its body is coated with blue glaze.
Its two sides are separately painted with a fan
with orchids on it. The jar was used for storing
medicine.

Preserved in Shaanxi Museum of Medical History

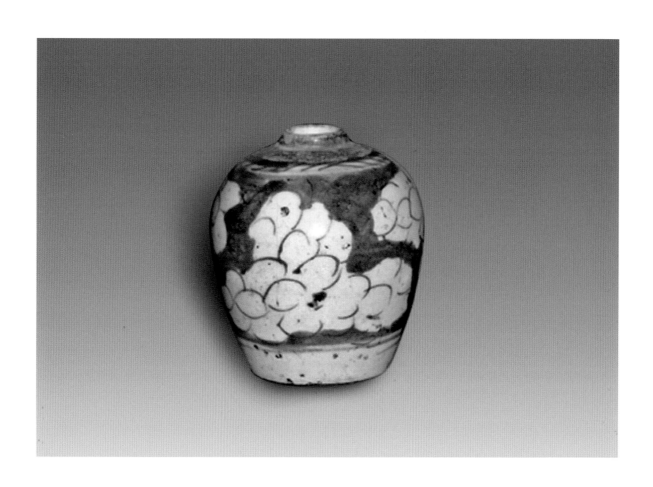

瓷药罐

清

瓷质

口径 2.5 厘米，底径 4.8 厘米，通高 8.8 厘米，重 200 克

Porcelain Medicine Jar

Qing Dynasty

Porcelain

Mouth Diameter 2.5 cm/ Bottom Diameter 4.8 cm/ Height 8.8 cm/ Weight 200 g

子母口，圆肩，圆腹，圈足。通体饰蓝底白
花图。盛贮器。

陕西医史博物馆藏

The jar has a snap-lid, a round shoulder, a round
belly and a ring foot. Its body is decorated
with patterns of white flowers on the blue
background. The jar was used for storing
medicine.

Preserved in Shaanxi Museum of Medical History

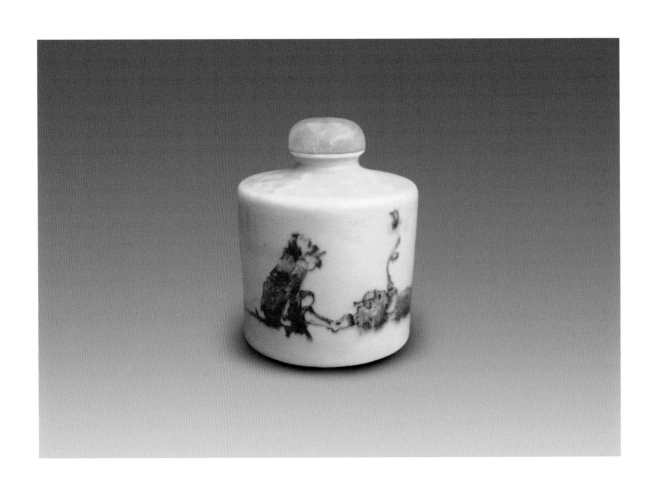

青花龙纹圆形药用盖罐

清

瓷质

腹径 9.7 厘米，通高 12 厘米，瓶身高 9.1 厘米，重 372 克

Round Medicine Bottle with Blue-and-white Dragon Patterns

Qing Dynasty

Porcelain

Belly Diameter 9.7 cm/ Height 12 cm/ Body Height 9.1 cm/ Weight 372 g

圆形短颈，口唇外突出，平底，带盖。器表彩绘医药人物。用于装药。

广东中医药博物馆藏

The round bottle has a lid, a protruded rim, a short neck and a flat bottom. Its surface is painted with colored patterns of medicine-related figures. The bottle was used for storing medicine.

Preserved in Guangdong Chinese Medicine Museum

索 引

（馆藏地按拼音字母排序）

Index

参考文献

[1] 李经纬 . 中国古代医史图录 [M]. 北京：人民卫生出版社，1992.

[2] 傅维康，李经纬，林昭庚 . 中国医学通史：文物图谱卷 [M]. 北京：人民卫生出版社，2000.

[3] 和中浚，吴鸿洲 . 中华医学文物图集 [M]. 成都：四川人民出版社，2001.

[4] 上海中医药博物馆 . 上海中医药博物馆馆藏珍品 [M]. 上海：上海科学技术出版社，2013.

[5] 西藏自治区博物馆 . 西藏博物馆 [M]. 北京：五洲传播出版社，2005.

[6] 崔乐泉 . 中国古代体育文物图录：中英文本 [M]. 北京：中华书局，2000.

[7] 张金明，陆雪春 . 中国古铜镜鉴赏图录 [M]. 北京：中国民族摄影艺术出版社，2002.

[8] 文物精华编辑委员会 . 文物精华 [M]. 北京：文物出版社，1964.

[9] 谭维四 . 湖北出土文物精华 [M]. 武汉：湖北教育出版社，2001.

[10] 常州市博物馆 . 常州文物精华 [M]. 北京：文物出版社，1998.

[11] 镇江博物馆 . 镇江文物精华 [M]. 合肥：黄山书社，1997.

[12] 贵州省文化厅，贵州省博物馆 . 贵州文物精华 [M]. 贵阳：贵州人民出版社，2005.

[13] 徐良玉 . 扬州馆藏文物精华 [M]. 南京：江苏古籍出版社，2001.

[14] 昭陵博物馆，陕西历史博物馆 . 昭陵文物精华 [M]. 西安：陕西人民美术出版社，1991.

[15] 南通博物苑 . 南通博物苑文物精华 [M]. 北京：文物出版社，2005.

[16] 邯郸市文物研究所 . 邯郸文物精华 [M]. 北京：文物出版社，2005.

[17] 张秀生，刘友恒，聂连顺，等 . 中国河北正定文物精华 [M]. 北京：文化艺术出版社，1998.

[18] 陕西省咸阳市文物局 . 咸阳文物精华 [M]. 北京：文物出版社，2002.

[19] 安阳市文物管理局 . 安阳文物精华 [M]. 北京：文物出版社，2004.

[20] 深圳市博物馆 . 深圳市博物馆文物精华 [M]. 北京：文物出版社，1998.

[21]《中国文物精华》编辑委员会 . 中国文物精华（1993）[M]. 北京：文物出版社，1993.

[22] 夏路，刘永生.山西省博物馆馆藏文物精华[M].太原：山西人民出版社，1999.

[23] 文物精华编辑委员会.文物精华[M].文物出版社，1957.

[24] 山西博物院，湖北省博物馆.荆楚长歌：九连墩楚墓出土文物精华[M].太原：山西人民出版社，2011.

[25] 刘广堂，石金鸣，宋建忠.晋国雄风：山西出土两周文物精华[M].沈阳：万卷出版公司，2009.

[26] 沈君山，王国平，单迎红.滦平博物馆馆藏文物精华[M].北京：中国文联出版社，2012.

[27] 张家口市博物馆.张家口市博物馆馆藏文物精华[M].北京：科学出版社，2011.

[28] 浙江省文物考古研究所.浙江考古精华[M].北京：文物出版社，1999.

[29] 故宫博物院.故宫雕刻珍萃[M].北京：紫禁城出版社，2004.

[30] 故宫博物院紫禁城出版社.故宫博物院藏宝录[M].上海：上海文艺出版社，1986.

[31] 首都博物馆.大元三都[M].北京：科学出版社，2016.

[32] 新疆维吾尔自治区博物馆.新疆出土文物[M].北京：文物出版社，1975.

[33] 王兴伊，段逸山.新疆出土涉医文书辑校[M].上海：上海科学技术出版社，2016.

[34] 刘学春.刍议医药卫生文物的概念与分类标准[J].中华中医药杂志，2016，31（11）:4406-4409.

[35] 上海古籍出版社.中国艺海[M].上海：上海古籍出版社，1994.

[36] 紫都，岳鑫.一生必知的200件国宝[M].呼和浩特：远方出版社，2005.

[37] 谭维四.湖北出土文物精华[M].武汉：湖北教育出版社，2001.

[38] 张建青.青海彩陶收藏与鉴赏[M].北京：中国文史出版社，2007.

[39] 银景琦.仡佬族文物[M].南宁：广西人民出版社，2014.

[40] 廖果，梁峻，李经纬.东西方医学的反思与前瞻[M].北京：中医古籍出版社，2002.

[41] 梁峻，张志斌，廖果，等.中华医药文明史集论[M].北京：中医古籍出版社，2003.

[42] 郑蓉，庄乾竹，刘聪，等.中国医药文化遗产考论[M].北京：中医古籍出版社，2005.